# IN SEARCH OF A MATCH

## Black & White

**By**

**Mr. Dan Moore, Sr.**

ISBN 1451520972  EAN-13 9781451520972.

All proceeds from this book support Marrow for Life, Inc.
A Georgia nonprofit 501 (c) (3) corporation

www.MarrowForLife.org

Dedicated to

Greek Gray and LaChandra Moore

Rod Gunn, Stacy Toney and Tina Saadat
Of Be the Match, whose dedication and tireless efforts are
helping to save lives.

Erma Hightower, a true inspiration
Cherie Fairfax, an overcomer
Taylor John, an inspiring young lady
Joyce Washington and Suzanne Gordon, Co-Founders of the
FACE Foundation, Inc.


And to all the patients, families and
Health Care Providers of those suffering with life threatening
diseases.

Special Thanks to

Ariel Howard,  Michele Mitchell, Estella Moore,
JaMika Witherspoon (JamPoet), Barbara Rigsby, Dee Robinson,
April Stevens, Sarita Thomas  and Lisa Wright

# Table of Contents

# THE AWAKENING

The weather was unseasonably mild on that February evening. I was shooting a documentary on Black Inventors at the APEX Museum in Atlanta. After the last take as we were about to wrap up, a charming young lady came into the APEX. At first glance she appeared to be in her early twenties.

She slipped into a seat and sat quietly observing me interviewing a young lady who was an inventor. During one of the breaks she introduced herself as Greek Gray. I then knew that this was the young lady I was expecting. She was here in Atlanta to undergo treatment for leukemia at an area hospital. She was eager to know more about the documentary we were shooting. When I explained to her it was about Black inventors, she seemed very interested. I asked if she wanted to participate. Without hesitation she asked what she could do. I replied "Just take a seat in front of the camera and talk about what you know about Black inventors and inventions."

She smiled warmly and took the seat. After she was properly set up and the camera was rolling, I asked her a few questions. Although shy, she immediately immersed herself into the scene and began to answer questions.

When we were finished, she came to me and began asking about the project, the APEX museum and its mission. After a few moments she expressed that she was a little tired and needed to go get some rest before going for her treatment.

She would later share her story with me. A story that would reveal to me how little I knew about leukemia. Greek Gray's story, changed my life and altered my path.

Here was a beautiful young lady in her thirties, appearing to be in her twenties and seemingly in good health, obviously in good spirits.

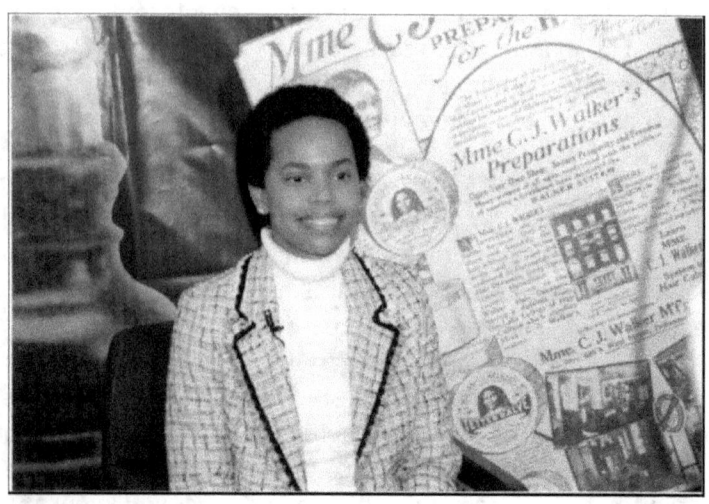

**Greek Gray visiting APEX Museum 2006**

The following week my wife and I visited her in the hospital. I then learned that she was here in Atlanta seeking treatment and hoping to find a marrow donor match. Although lying in the hospital bed, she was still the charming and personable person I had met earlier. She was very gracious and considerate.

We asked if there was anything we could bring her or do for her. She thanked us and said she was fine. Even after persistence, she still accepted our offer but graciously said there was nothing she needed. We then talked to her friend who accompanied her to Atlanta and was looking after her. With reluctance she said,

"Well the food here is O Kay but I know that she would love to have some vegetarian food."

On our next visit we were able to find a vegetarian food store and bring her some of her favorites. Her smile and appreciation were atypical of who she was - a very kind and gentle spirit.

Her dilemma, I later learned, began in 2004. She was a fitness training and sports writer, seemingly in good health. She was not feeling well one day and went to see the doctor. After being tested she learned that she had Acute Myelogenous Leukemia (AML)

She underwent treatment and received a marrow transplant and was in remission. After a period of time she relapsed. Now, her best and perhaps only chance was to find a willing marrow donor that would be a match.

Then the search began. I made contact with Rod Gunn of the National Marrow Donor Program (NMDP) now called Be The Match Registry, who later introduced me to his colleague, Stacy Toney. Rod and Stacy, were two very dedicated individuals working as recruiters for the NMDP. Their territory was all of Georgia and parts of Alabama. I found it difficult to believe they were responsible for such a large territory on such an important mission. They were responsible for recruiting donors from the African American community to help fill a void in the national donor registry.

Then the hard cold facts began to come to life. I discovered that there were more than seven million donors on the registry and only eight percent were Black. Because most, but not all, marrow transplants are race specific, the chance of an African American finding a match is very rare.

Equipped with this knowledge, I immediately began to work with Rod and Stacy to organize drives to recruit donors. I pulled together a group of interested persons and formed a non-profit corporation called Marrow For Life. The first year we worked with Rod and Stacy we were able to register more than eight hundred new donors on the registry.

The fire was ignited and many people began to get involved. Jo Roberson Edwards arranged a donor drive at the Phyllis Wheatly YWCA which was covered by Tiffany Cochran of WXIA TV. Dee Robinson and her singing group, Black Pearls, held a drive at The APEX Museum. Donor drives were also held at area churches including St. Phillip AME, New Birth Missionary Baptist and others. Sister Girlfriends, a group of nurses and medical technicians joined the effort along with others. There were accountants like Lisa Wright, aroma therapists, Sarita Thomas and international recording artist, Jean Carne. Camille Russell Love of the City of Atlanta's Bureau of Cultural Affairs arranged a drive at the Atlanta Jazz Festival and people from all walks of life began to see the need and join the effort. My wife, Estella set up a web page and there was an outpouring of love, compassion and support. Erskine Hawkins of the Georgia Black United Fund began to help this new organization, Marrow for Life, and position us for funding from corporate and government sources.

Meanwhile, Greek Gray was battling her illness. She was being a real trooper and even attended one of the donor drives. But the hope was beginning to fade. Time was running out.

Greek Gray – *"I had a promising career as an American Council on Exercise (ACE) Certified Fitness Trainer, Nutrition Specialist, and Contributing Health and Fitness Writer. On my 33rd birthday while functioning as founder and president of the Las Vegas-based GKG Fitness Company training many affluent singles on exercise and nutrition to achieve optimum health and fitness, I was diagnosed with Acute Myelogenous Leukemia (AML) in 2004."*

*"I am 34 years old and my leukemia went into remission prior to my stem cell bone marrow transplant at the University of California Los Angeles (UCLA) Hospital Transplant Center back on May 3, 2005."*

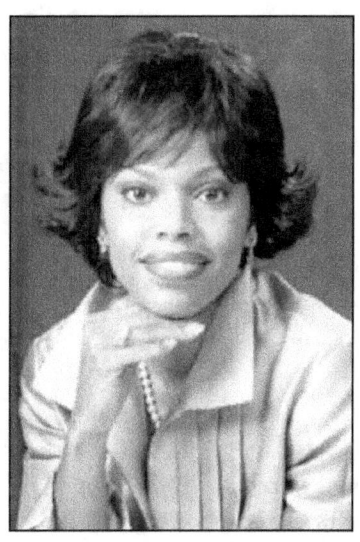

**Greek Gray**
August 26, 1971-August 14, 2006

*"At the time I would have been considered one of the lucky blood cancer victims because the Oncology specialist determined that I was a candidate to become my own stem-cell bone marrow transplant donor due to my health condition, lifestyle and medical history."*

*"Since using your own stem cell transplant is not a cure those who suffer with leukemia and other blood related diseases have death sentences that are depending on a bone marrow transplant from a sibling and/or an unrelated donor for survival."*

*"I thank God the cancer has not killed me, but around me in the hospital many others were not so fortunate. My fight is not just with me anymore. It is for others afflicted with leukemia that will be able to be served by the Greek Gray Leukemia Foundation. I know that my foundation can't save the world or for that matter cover every aspect of our state of health in this society, but my foundation can become the catalyst behind nationwide drives in churches, community based centers and organizations to seek bone marrow donors needed so others can have a second chance at life!"*

Following my first meeting with Greek I penned these words.
***"I have only met you once. But then, one only has to meet you once, to feel your warm and gentle spirit."***

*You are...*
Gracious
Radiant
Empowering
Elegant
Kind and loving

At 1 am August 14, 2006, Greek Gray made her transition.

During one of our Marrow for Life planning meetings, Rod Gunn invited a patient with whom he was working. The moment will ever be indelibly impressed in my memory. Two ladies came to the meeting. They were mother and daughter, but looked more like sisters. It was Rosie Ivey and her daughter LaChandra Moore. Tears filled the eyes of most of us present as LaChandra began to tell her story. She was a 26 year old single mother of three boys, age eight, ten and twelve.

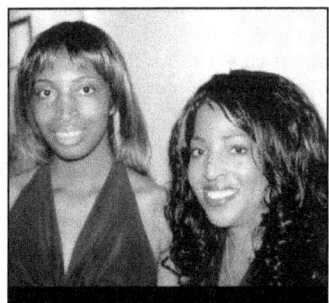

**LaChandra Moore and Rosie Ivey**

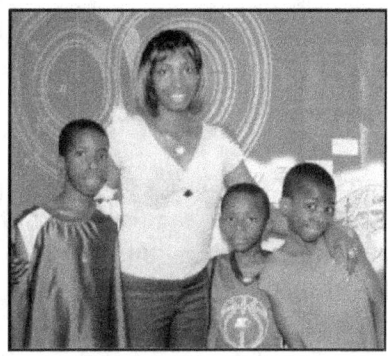

**LaChandra Moore, Isaac, Ameer and Nigel**

Her story is perhaps like the stories of many others diagnosed with leukemia. She was working for a medical records firm. She had headaches occasionally but no other signs of a serious illness. One day at work she became dizzy and passed out. She was taken to the hospital. Then came the shock of her life. The doctor informed her that she had leukemia. It was February 14th, Valentine's Day, and this was her news. Her first thoughts were of her three boys. She thought perhaps there was a wrong diagnosis. Maybe the medical reports were mixed up. Then reality set in. She had leukemia, a life threatening blood cancer.

After hearing her story the reaction was the same with everyone. We had to do more. We had to step up our efforts. Put on more drives. Recruit more Blacks for the national registry. Another challenge was before us. Not a number or statistic, but a person, a family in need.

LaChandra's mother Rosie had just moved to Atlanta from California. So at least there was a support system in place. The months that followed were challenging. It was chemo therapy with all its adverse side effects. There were three boys that had to get back and forth to school and now two houses to maintain.

As the search continued for a donor match various experimental drugs were tested. However, to no avail. And then there was finally a break. They found a match. LaChandra and Rosie were elated. At last, a real glimmer of hope. There were three matches found during the search. And then the tragedy struck. They were unable to find two of the donors. They were placed on the registry sometime ago but had moved without notifying the NMDP and there was no way to locate them. Despite the fact that donors were asked to notify the national Marrow Donor Program if they moved or changed their mind, they had failed to do so. The third donor changed their mind.

It is difficult to imagine the let down and total frustration when the three potential donors were not found or had changed their mind. How did LaChandra feel after having her hopes raised only to have them crash? What went through Rosie's mind when the hope for her daughter's recovery was shattered? It only further emphasizes the importance of really being committed to help save a life, anyone's life - not just a person that you may know who had leukemia and was your reason for registering.

As LaChandra's condition began to worsen, my wife and I made several trips to the hospital. While she visited with Lachandra and Rosie, I stayed in the waiting room, unable to bare seeing her suffer.

And then one night the dreaded phone call came. LaChandra Moore made her transition. Rosie while looking through LaChandra's Bible after she passed she found this hand written note from her 12 year old son Isaac.

"Lord please wash away all my momma's cancer cells & get her a bone marrow transplant"
Love you

# THE DRIVES
# AND
# THE DRIVERS

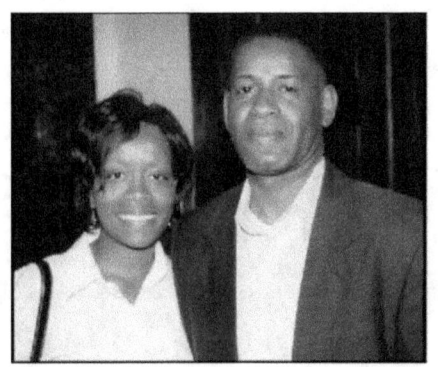

**Stacy Toney & Rod Gunn**
**Recruiters**
National Marrow Donor Program (NMDP)
Be The Match

It is often a challenge to get people to register to become a marrow donor. This is particularly true in the Black community. For some, there is a fear of the unknown or misconceptions and misinformation regarding the negative effects it will have on them. Others are distrustful recalling such incidents as the Tuskegee experiment and other forms of clinical tests that had negative effects.

There is a shortage of donors from the African American community on the national register. Most marrow transplants are race specific. With more than 7 million on the national register, only 8% are Black, this severely decreases the chances that a Black person with leukemia, will find a match.

The Black church is one of the most vital places to conduct donor drives. Here in Georgia there are two very dedicated individuals who serve as recruiters for the National Marrow Donor Program. Rod Gunn and Stacy Toney are responsible for all of Georgia and parts of Alabama. With a territory this large, it is difficult to manage this task without a group of dedicated volunteers. Despite this enormous task, Rod and Stacy work tirelessly to meet the challenge of enrolling Blacks on the registry.

Rod and Stacy are the drivers that keep the drives going. Sometimes recruiting as many as five hundred donors in one location, they have an overwhelming task and responsibility.

Rod Gunn has been with the marrow donor program since 2004. He discusses his most challenging and rewarding moments.
" The most challenging part of my job is adding enough Blacks and African Americans onto the registry to make a significant difference in the percentage of Black  patients who can find a matching donor to give them the lifesaving marrow or blood stem cell transplant they need to cure them of their disease. Only 17% of Black patients receive a transplant within the first 6-months of diagnosis. Since tissue type is hereditary, like eye

color, a patient is more likely to match a donor of the same racial or ethnic background. As a result, we need to add millions of Blacks onto the marrow donor registry to give Black patients a better chance of finding a lifesaving donor."

Rod recalls his most memorable encounters. "My most rewarding experience(s) are those occasions where I've been able to contribute to changing the mindset of potential Black donors who previously refused to join the marrow donor registry because of rumors or misinformation. After properly educating people with the facts about joining the marrow donor registry, it's amazing to see that many are willing to participate."

Stacy Toney often talks about her biggest challenges and rewards. "My most discouraging experiences have been the many occasions where I've attended the funeral of Black patients who didn't receive the lifesaving transplant they needed." Rod also recalls his most memorable encounters. "My most rewarding experience(s) are those occasions where I've been able to contribute to changing the mindset of potential Black donors who previously refused to join the marrow donor registry because of rumors or misinformation. After properly educating people with the facts about joining the marrow donor registry, it's amazing to see that many are willing to participate."

" My role with the National Marrow Donor Program is to bring about awareness and education in our communities about the need for more marrow and blood stem cell donors and particularly in the African American community. "

"We like to work with captured groups, but anytime we can get to people, and let them know that there is a need for more donors, we will be there."

"I know there's a need, and I get my reward when I'm helping people, because that is my gift. That is one of the purposes God has me here to help people. But it's in my heart and I'm very passionate about it and I know how it can change someone's life. I know that if someone can get a match, and that match works well, someone can be given back their child. Someone can have back their mother. Someone can have back their best friend."

"I get the calls every day and that drives me even more when I know it's someone's father, someone's best friend, someone's cousin and they are desperate. They need a match or they feel like it's a death sentence if they don't get that match. And for some people it is. I've seen some people come in and look for a match, and look for a match, and look for a match and not find that match and pass away when I know there are people out there that may be a match. We just have to get them educated, and then they can make a decision to join the registry."

"We ask people to be responsible. We ask if you join the registry, and you decide later that your commitment needs to change for whatever reason, call us and let us know. We will take you off the registry, no questions asked. But as long as people are on the registry it is important that they take their commitment seriously, because someone's life is on the other end, and that person doesn't have the luxury of backing out. They need you. They need someone to save their life, and if you match someone, really how could you say no to someone's life? We know that if we or someone we know were in need, we would not want someone to say no to our life."

"We used to take a small blood sample. Now all it takes is a simple swab of the jaw to place you on the registry. We do extensive screenings to make sure it's safe for the donor and the recipient. Marrow is what's within your bones. It contains cells that make blood. They make your red blood cells, your white blood cells, and your platelets. People that have diseases like leukemia or sickle cell anemia need these transplants. Their blood forming cells, we call them blood stem cells, are not doing what they need to do, and that person is deteriorating in health. If their white blood cells are not doing what they are supposed to do, they can't fight off infections like healthy people. If their red blood cells aren't doing what they're supposed to do they are lethargic. They're tired. They don't have enough energy to carry on with their normal daily activities. If their platelet count is low, then when they bleed they just keep bleeding and not stop. Platelets are some of the factors that help you stop bleeding. When people bruise a lot that means they're bleeding under their skin, so these people need healthy marrow from people like you or me to be able to live a functional life. And the great thing about it is anybody between the ages of 18 and 60, in general good health, not even perfect health, just general good health, usually have good bone marrow and can donate to someone and save a life."

Stacy continues, "Now personally, I got on the registry about ten years ago when one of my sorority sisters needed a transplant. We were in college and we all thought that maybe we would be a match so we all signed up. It's a serious thing. We must recognize that if you get on the registry you may never be called. I haven't been called yet and it has been about ten years. But I'm committed to go through whatever is necessary to save someone's life until my 61st birthday, and I've got quite a way to go. "

"When we (NMDP) first organized and staffed donor drives it required a blood sample to register. Now, with new technology all that is needed is a cheek swab test. From this, a person could be listed on the registry and available for a patient if there is a match.

With this new technology came a new opportunity. I knew that individuals desiring to get on the registry had to search for a time and place where a drive was taking place. With only two recruiters covering all of Georgia and parts of Alabama, it was virtually impossible to accommodate all those wanting to join the registry. As a start I persuaded the regional Manager of the NMDP to allow the APEX Museum to be an official testing site. Armed with this, we began aggressively recruiting donors to visit the APEX on the day we were officially not open (Mondays) and be able to register. The APEX (African American Panoramic Experience) became the first official testing site in Georgia to accommodate potential donor registration.

It is abundantly clear that volunteers play a vital role. We then set up a training manual and power point presentation to assist Rod and Stacy in recruiting volunteers. Their enthusiasm was infectious. Volunteers were trained and began to help in many of the donor drives. In our first year we registered more than 800 people. That number may be small but hopefully it will provide a matching donor for someone in need.

In addition to church drives, shopping malls, college campuses and health fairs provide opportunities for recruitment efforts. It is also an opportunity for fraternities, sororities, clubs and social organizations to provide a great community service by having their members participate in donor drives.

The thorough training provided by Rod and Stacy, I have come to realize, is so crucial. One of the things they continue to emphasize to those registering, "If you change your mind, please notify the NMDP and ask to be removed from the registry. You will remove you from the registry, no questions asked." This is so important. A patient having gone through rigorous treatment may be notified that a match has been found. This elevates the hope for the patient and their family. If the potential donor then changes their mind, it can prove devastating to the patient and their family.

Rod and Stacy also stress in their training, the importance of giving accurate information on the primary address of the donor but also a good alternative address. It is important to notify the NMDP if there is a change of address. If the donor is called upon and cannot be located, it is again a devastating experience for the patient and their family.

Sometime donors come forth and register because they have a friend or loved one with leukemia, sickle cell anemia or other disorder and in dire need of a transplant. If that friend or loved one receives successful treatment or if they pass, the donor in some cases, does not wish to be considered for someone else. Again, it is important to remove your name from the registry to avoid disappointing a patient in need.

The donor giving accurate and complete information before they commit is imperative. It helps assure the donor bank is populated with viable donors willing to help save a life, anyone's.

## Donor Drives

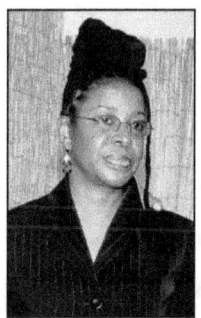 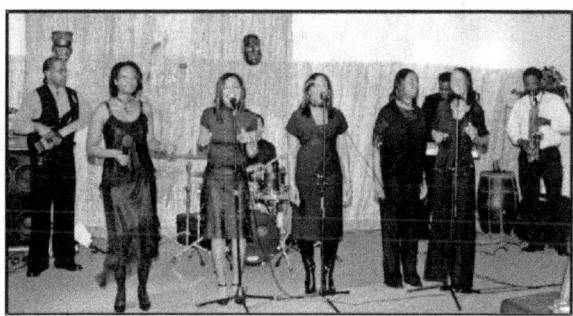

**Dee Robinson and The Black Pearls @ APEX Donor Drive**

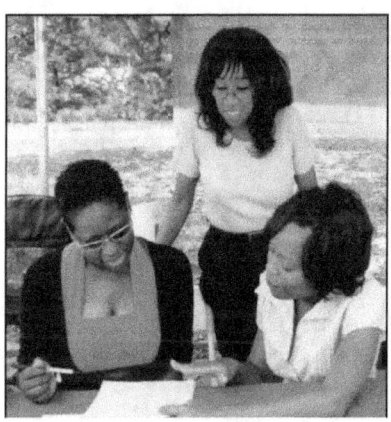

**International Recording Artist, Jean Carne, Candace Anderson, and Stacy Toney @APEX Drive Atlanta Jazz Festival**

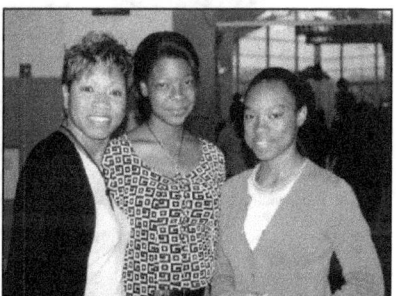

**Sarita Thomas and daughters Mya Thomas (age 18), Sadivia Wilson (age 16)**

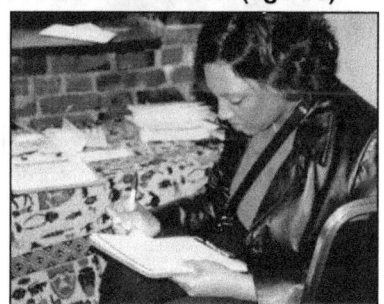

**LaTrice of Sister Girlfriends Prepares for APEX Drive**

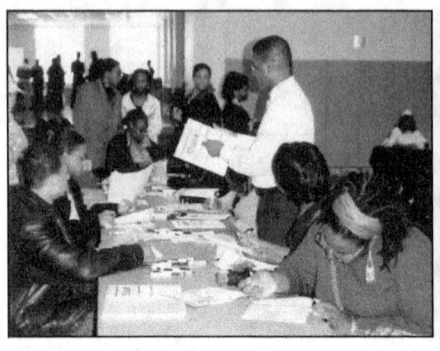

**Rod Gunn**
**New Birth Missionary Baptist**

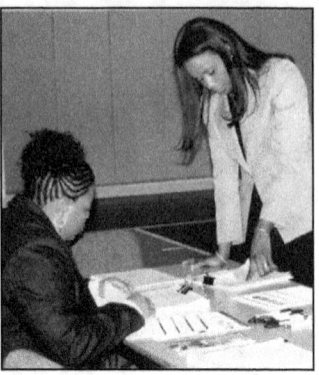

**Erma Hightower**
**(standing)**

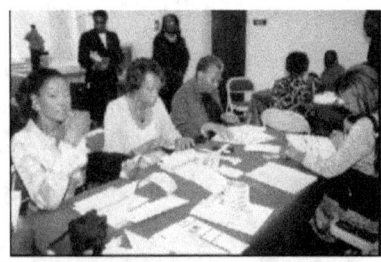

**St. Phillip AME Church**

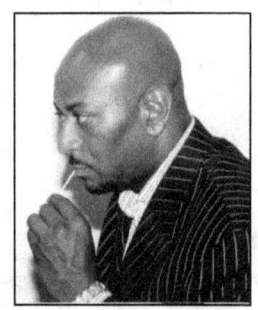

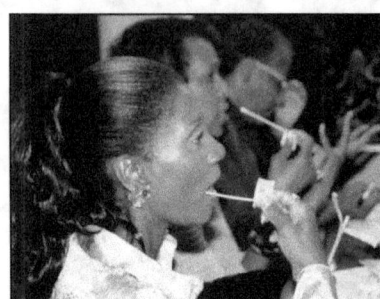

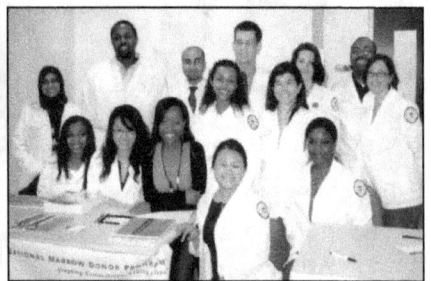

**Pharmacy students from**
**Mercer University**

Volunteer Sarita Thomas, tells of her involvement.

"I believe that we were all created with the purpose to serve mankind. My constant prayer is that GOD aligns me with the people and places I am to serve. My journey with Marrow for Life began with a phone call from a very wise man. Dan Moore Sr., called and asked if I would be a available to sit in on a discussion group for a project he would like to take flight. After a brief introduction on the subject of the need of bone marrow donations in the Black community I was sure that this was my calling! I attended several round table discussions and training sessions for preparation to participate as a volunteer. This experience has changed my life! In the beginning I found that I was not qualified to be a donor due to problems associated with a back injury-but I was able to be a volunteer! I am now able to be a part of the giving and receiving of life's love and continuous joy! I can help my fellow man gain the knowledge and fulfillment of the gift of life! I have traveled to many locations to teach and recruit donors and volunteers. I have introduced my teenaged stepchildren and their friends to Marrow for Life as volunteers and they assist me with donor drives (and love doing so). During this time I was blessed to conceive and deliver my first child and was overjoyed to be able to donate my umbilical cord! The greatest opportunity to see GOD at work is to meet and share with those in need of donations. The desire to continue forward in this life with the blessing of optimum health has great meaning to them. Their stories have given me so much HOPE and DETERMINATION to continue forward spreading the message of the Importance of bone marrow donation!"

One of our volunteers, Dee Robinson, responded to the call and attended some of our preliminary meetings. She decided to do her part by having a singing group that she manages perform at The APEX and invite guests to attend and sign up to be marrow donors.

When the performance was about to begin, I remember very vividly having the unpleasant task of announcing the person they were coming to support, LaChandra Moore, had only days before lost her battle. As they sang their opening number I was moved to tears when I thought, at that very hour LaChandra's family was in Mississippi laying her to rest. It punctuated the fact that there had to be escalated efforts to get more African American donors on the marrow registry.

Dee Robinson, author and promoter shares her commitment and passion.

"Why I Care. I frequently visit the APEX Museum in Atlanta, and I have learned of many historical events, particularly about African Americans in Atlanta. During one visit, there was a display showing the disparity in the number of African Americans in need of bone marrow transplants and the number of African Americans donors.

From that display I learned that for a transplant to be successful, the donor and the recipient's marrow must be the same genetic type. Simply meaning, the possibility for a match is only possible if the donor and the recipient are of the same ethnic group, with rare exception.

I didn't know that. In addition, I figured there were enough donors for everyone in need, so the matter would take care of itself. That is not the case.

I'm empathetic by nature, so I often ask myself, "What if it were me?"

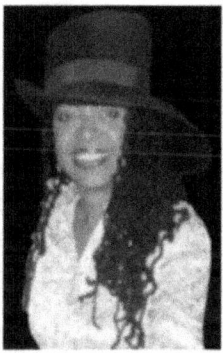

Dee Robinson

If I were in need of assistance, I would want someone to be there for me. So, for me, my involvement with bone marrow donation awareness campaign is reflective of the Golden Rule: *Do unto others as you would have them do unto you.*

I am sensitive to the concerns of others and find it difficult to be emotionally distant to someone who is suffering. I will do whatever I can to help alleviate their pain and suffering. The fact of the matter is that we need each other. There have been no sociological advancements without people being concerned about each other. I see helping others in need just as much of a social concern as is voting.

For leukemia and other blood borne diseases, a bone marrow transplant is considered the only real cure. That's when reality set in for me – if I was unaware of this problem, there are probably a lot of other people like me who might be propelled into action if they only knew. I believe that lack of awareness and information are the main reasons that African American donors are under-represented on the national registries.

I strongly believe in people helping people, the village raising the child, each one teaching one, and so on. I felt compelled to do something to get the word out to the community about the need for more African American donors.

One of our awareness events included a speaker presenting the facts and live entertainment, followed by the attendees signing up to become potential donors. This type of event can hopefully become a regularly recurring format to disseminate information about the dire need for African American bone marrow donors.

One of my favorite African proverbs says it best: *I am because we are, and because we are, therefore I am.* ~~ Aşe (Amen)

One of the most incredible drives that I have witnessed was organized by 10 year old Pat Padraja. Pat's story is unique and awe inspiring.

"I was diagnosed with Acute Lymphoblastic Leukemia in March 2006. This diagnosis came after a long, painful year suffering from what we then thought was Juvenile Rheumatoid Arthritis. The pain and swelling in my joints got so bad that I was in a wheelchair for 5 months because I was unable to walk a single step. When the pain got worse and I had a fever that wouldn't go away my doctors put me in the hospital where they found out that I really have Leukemia. I am undergoing chemotherapy treatments at St. Josephs Children's Hospital in Tampa, Florida and will continue those treatments until July 2009."

"I live near Tampa, Florida with my mom, Claudine, stepdad, Keith, two brothers, Nathan, (12) and Tucker, (6), my sister Jocelyn and my beloved Bulldog, Rinkles. My dad, William, lives in South Florida."

" I love sports, especially hockey and baseball! I can't play hockey or baseball right now because of the Leukemia and that makes me sad but I love going to see games! I have to be careful because my immune system is weak and I can't get hurt because that could be dangerous for me if my platelets are low. I also am a straight A student and really like history."

" I heard about the shortage of bone marrow donors especially for minority groups, when a friend of mine died because she couldn't find a matching donor. That made me so sad and I want to do something to help! I am part Hispanic, and am scared that if I need a bone marrow transplant one day there may not be a match available for me."

"I am excited to plan and organize DRIVING FOR DONORS and

I hope you will help me. It is scary because it is such a large task but I can do it with your help!"

This, keep in mind, is from a young man only ten years old. Pat brought his campaign to Atlanta. It was most impressive. Pat set a goal on his national tour to register 2008 new donors. He registered more than 5000. Pat later went on to receive an award on CNN for his courageous work.

Pat's mother, Claudine, expressed her pride in her son for taking on such a enormous task. She tells how Pat while planning his first local tour went to bed and awoke the next morning to announce he wanted to take the tour nationally.

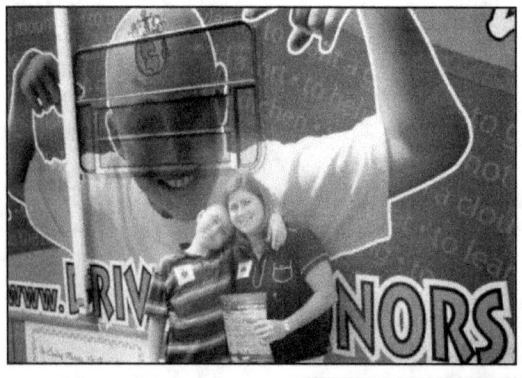

**Pat and his mother Claudine hold donor drive at The APEX Museum.**

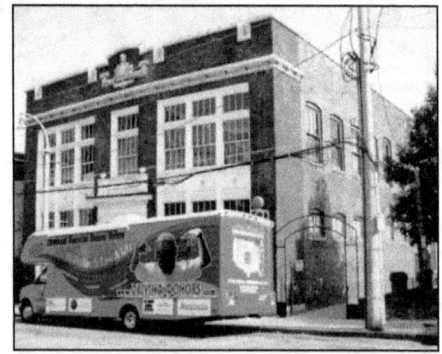

Michele Mitchell, Gallery coordinator for the APEX Museum, tells of her experience. "For quite some time I'd hear about the marrow donor program and would say I would register but would never really put the effort into it. I was heading to work a couple of years ago and I was listening to a talk radio station. They were talking about how important it is for Black people to join the registry.

I learned something that morning that really pushed me to respond. I learned that this was something that was race specific. I give blood regularly, But I don't recall anyone ever asking me to be a marrow donor or about the importance to patients with blood disorders. I learned that the chances for people of color to survive are very slim compared to those other races. That really made me feel I had an obligation to go to the drive and register. But I wasn't necessarily turning my car in the direction of the West End Mall where the drive was being held. At that point I thought that maybe I'll go during lunch or I'll make a point of doing it later on some other time, but then they said something else. They really told me how simple and quick it would be, and they made it so that you really could not refuse to go. Every excuse I had in my head about why I couldn't go at that moment they squashed for me. Excuses like well it'll take me too long to get there, by the time I get there, I'll be late for work, etc... But really it was close to where I worked, within ten minutes.] So the drive wasn't that bad. It was also a process I could have gone through pretty fast, in about 30 minutes and I would have been on my way back to work on time or maybe just a few minutes late. I would have been able to accomplish it, so they really made it very convenient. They made it so that I would have felt really, really bad had I not gone that morning. They took away every excuse that existed and made me feel like it was necessary that as a person [and] as a human being, and as an African American that this was my obligation and I could not turn my back on it then."

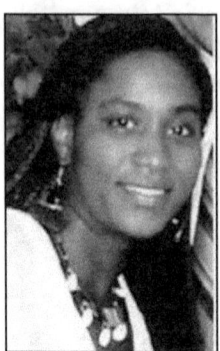

**Michele Mitchell**

"One was the pain. Bone marrow is in the bone. That's all I ever associated with; you know, something going inside of my bone, holes drilling inside bone, which is not a pleasant thought. So the pain would keep me from it and thinking [about] would I really want to do this. Is this something that I can go through? I give blood, I give plasma, that's simple, that's easy so that was my counter for it. Okay, I might not be a bone marrow donor but I donate all these other things. But [it was] the pain that I thought was involved with it really kept me from doing it. But once I was able to go that day and see some of the films, I learned [that there are] different methods of donating bone marrow. So you didn't really have to be afraid of somebody going into your bone, and the pain associated with it anymore, because you had other options. So that made it simpler."

I think most people are probably like me: we just don't have the right information. Normally when the person has the right information, as a human being no matter what race, you see the obligation that you have, and it really is not a choice. It's something that we ought to do as people. Whether you have had the opportunity to save someone's life, or someone has saved your life, it's something that we all ought to do. I mean if we're here our life is a gift, and if a few moments of your time or a couple of your blood cells can save someone's life I don't see how any human being could say no. "

Volunteer Candace Skinner, shares her experience. "I became a volunteer at the APEX Museum in May 2003. Initially I worked in the gallery as a greeter. I enjoyed the experience and the atmosphere. I learned that in addition to being a historical site, The APEX under the leadership of its founding president, Dan Moore, Sr., had taken on various community projects. One of these projects was recruiting marrow donors for the national registry."

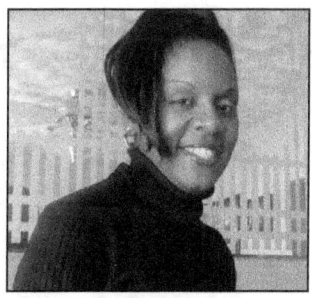

**Candace Skinner**

"A marrow drive was scheduled and they were short of volunteers to assist. I volunteered to accompany Mr. Moore to the drive. It was being held for employees of a day care center. As I learned more about the need for Blacks on the registry I was faced with a decision. After assisting in a drive I felt a sense of urgency to "Help Save a Life" through joining the registry. After all, how could I recruit others, if I was not willing to join? "

"I have been on the registry since December 2006. On April 29, 2009 I received a letter from The National Marrow Donor Program suggesting I was a potential match for someone in need of a transplant. My heart began to beat very fast. Surprised that signing the Registry was FOR REAL!! I called Buffalo, New York to share the news with my family and friends. Some could not believe me. I proceeded with the process by donating 5 Tubes of blood for testing and continuing to be a "Potential Match." I Interviewed by phone with a representative in Washington, D.C to walk me through the process. About 8 weeks later I received another letter stating that at this time, for some unknown reason, the patient was no longer In need of a transplant. I had mixed feelings I felt disappointed and relieved. I will still remain active in registering others to 'HELP SAVE A LIFE.' I know, now more than ever, the importance of not only being on the registry, but being available if ever you are called."

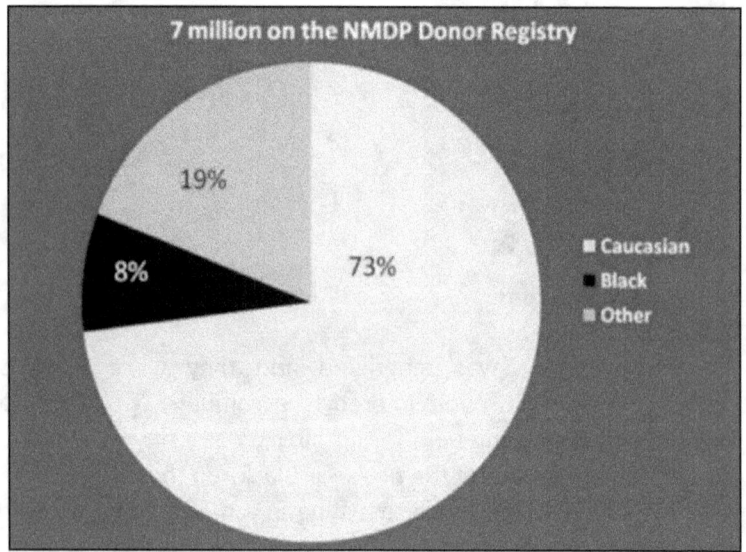

While most of the drives we conducted were to recruit marrow donors, we often set the stage for umbilical cord donation. In my research I learned that a very powerful option in the treatment of leukemia and sickle cell disease is the umbilical cord. Unfortunately, only a few states have public cord blood banks.

This is when I met Tina Saadat with a cord blood bank in Florida. She was stationed here in Atlanta and became a very active with the Marrow for Life project and arranged for the collection and facilitation of umbilical cords for public storage. unlike private storage which has an initial cost and annual maintenance fees, the public bank is usually free to the donor and is made available to anyone in need.

When I think about how many people could possibly be cured and how many umbilical cords are destroyed, it becomes unconscionable. I know of a cord that was called to save a patient's life that had been collected five years prior. This demonstrates the value of a life saving resource that is under-utilized.

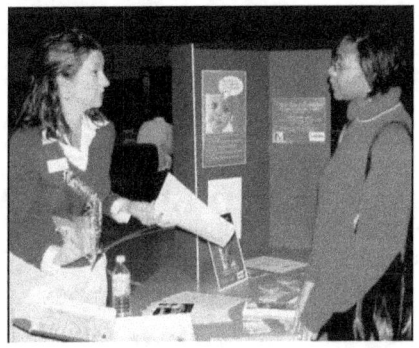 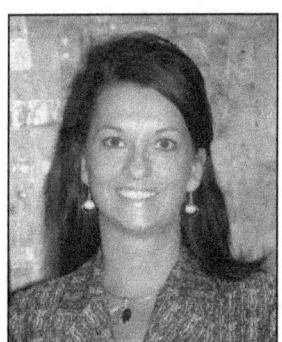

Tina Saadat explains cord donations

So we will push on to help establish and/or use public cord blood banks to help save lives.

I cannot help but reflect on the documentary I made some thirty=plus years ago. It is amazing to revisit this and witness the changes and yet, how many things remain the same, It is encouraging to know that Dr. Eckman had the vision to establish a Sickle Cell clinic at Grady Memorial Hospital which became the first in the nation with a 24.7 Emergency room.

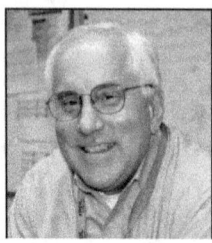

Dr. James Eckman
Dir. Sickle Cell Center
Grady Health Systems

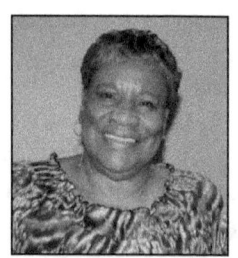

D. Jean Brannan, Pres.
Sickle Cell Foundation of
Georgia

I appreciate the work of the national and the local Sickle Cell Associations that continue to remind us about screening to prevent this life-threatening disease. This is perhaps one disease that we can wipe out in a number of years if testing was done so both parents could know the risks if they both have sickle cell trait.

During the interviews the message was consistent in praise for the Children's Health Care of Atlanta and Egleston Hospital for their compassion and competence in dealing with patients.

It is also rewarding to know about all the researchers and health care providers and organizations for their continued tireless efforts to bring a cure and hope to the patients and families they serve.

# THE DONORS

There are a myriad of myths and misconception regarding bone marrow donations. The recruiters often hear comments and are queried about the effects of being a bone marrow donor. This can best be answered by those who have been marrow donors for no one can tell the story better.

The questions span a spectrum and are mainly asked because of misinformation. "If I become a marrow donor, will I be crippled?" "Will I get leukemia if I am a donor?" "What are the risks to me if I am a marrow donor?" "I am told it is very painful. Will I be able to walk?"

I have had the opportunity to talk to several marrow donors. Although their experiences were different, there was one underlying factor. If asked if they would do it again, the answer was "yes", unanimously. "When it comes to saving someone's life I would do it all over again."

**Meet Erma Hightower**. She holds a full time job in a major law firm and is mother of five children. Erma has incredible faith and her loving and compassionate spirit is contagious.

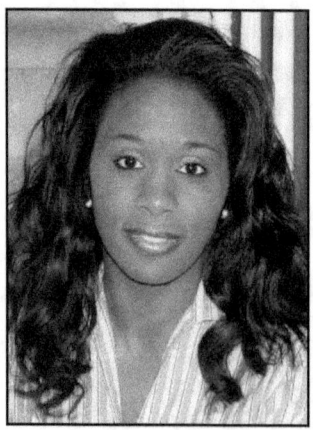

**Erma Hightower**

"In 2002, my husband was diagnosed with ---- He would need a marrow transplant. At that time I knew nothing about leukemia but only knew that my husband had to find a matching donor on the national registry. A few of my friends got together and organized bone marrow donor drives. I also signed up to become a donor."

"I was told that finding a matching donor was like finding a needle in a hay stack. But I knew that the Lord would help me find that needle. Several months later I received a phone call from the National Marrow Donor Program. The caller said,' Mrs. Hightower, we have searched the registry and you are a match for a 22 year old man.' I was shocked. Here my husband needed a transplant and I was a match for someone else. I pulled myself together and said 'Yes', I will do it."

"I began to prepare my mind for what was to come. I knew without a doubt that whatever it would take, I would definitely go through with it."

"And then several days later I received another call from the National Marrow Donor Program. This time the caller said to me, 'Mrs. Hightower, we have searched our donor base and we have located a matching donor for your husband.'" "I was simply overwhelmed and grateful that God had answered my prayers."

"As I prepared to become a donor for the 22 year old man, I was grateful that I was a match. To make sure I was in good health and that there would be no danger to me. I underwent a complete physical provided by the NMDP. When I checked out O Kay, I then went to the hospital to have my cells harvested. I remember talking to the doctor and the next thing I remember I heard the nurse saying, 'Wake up Mrs. Hightower, Wake up. You are our hero for the day.' The procedure went very smoothly. It was on a Friday and I was back to work that Monday. I was not in any severe pain but felt stiffness as though I had been exercising.

I have five children, and believe me the pain was not even to be compared, If I had it to do over again, I would, without hesitation. It is truly awesome to know that you were able to help save someone's life."

"I'm a mother of five, married, work full time and balancing life can be stressful but God allows me to endure. One of the things I've learned is, surround yourself with friends and family with positive advice when finding out about a life threatening disease."

Note: *Erma Hightower's husband did receive a transplant. He was doing fine, but several months later there were complications and he did not survive.*

**Meet Lummie LaShay Allen Harris-** She is an energetic librarian with a love for teaching and learning.

"I am originally from a small town in South Georgia called Portal. I got married and moved to Atlanta in 2000. I actually attempted to donate blood twice, but as you can tell, I'm pretty small in stature so I did not weigh enough. When I was in college I was participating with the blood drive that was associated with the National Marrow Donor Program. I was told even though I could not give blood, I could become a marrow donor. I said no problem. I asked about what pain was involved, but that wasn't a big issue so I signed on at that time, and that was back in 1993. I had totally, forgotten about it until I received a call. I believe it was in 2003. They tracked me down. Apparently I had some pretty good forwarding addresses, so they tracked my address to my parents home and they had my mother forward the information to me. So, that's how I initially found out that I was possibly a match for someone. But I had been on the registry for ten years before I received any contact."

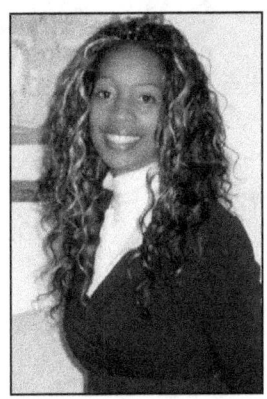

**Lummie Harris**

"I just always believed that no matter what, if there's something you can give of yourself that's actually free and doesn't cost anything, and it's actually going to save someone's life, then I don't see why not do it. To me it kind of baffles me when people give excuses about, 'well it's going to hurt, or I'm just not quite sure about it', and I also think possibly in the African American community it may be a little bit of just not knowing and not understanding. But sometimes when we don't know and we don't understand, we really need to research and look into it first other than just saying I don't know and just leaving it at that. For African Americans it is harder for us to find matches due to our genetics."

" My first thought was Wow, they kept up with that stuff. And honestly I didn't give it a second thought. I said if I'm a match, sure, why not. I remember when I was in college we found out that my niece had cancer.  We found out that it was terminal. It was a possibility that maybe we could donate bone marrow to save her life. So it was at that time that I said, if I ever can save someone's life I will. To experience someone, especially a young person, go through a terminal illness was heartbreaking. Ironically for me, the person that I ended up matching happened to be an infant. So, I just really believed that was my opportunity to do something for someone, something that unfortunately, I could not do for my niece. So when my mom called I said sure of course. My mother said, 'are you sure you want to do it?' My reply was yeah mom, I don't see why not. They were 100% behind me. They were still a little apprehensive but said go ahead if that's really what you want to do. I'm glad that I did have their blessing."

"My niece was five when we found out she had cancer. She was in kindergarten.  She had brain cancer, and it was in a place where it was inoperable."

"After I became a donor I was told that I could find out who the recipient was after a year, if I wanted to. That's the only thing that I have not wanted to do. I like to feel and know that I saved someone, even if it was just for a moment or a few days, weeks, months or years. I just like to hope that I did give them the opportunity to be with their loved ones for a longer period of time. I also like to think that they're still with us now. If they ever wanted to find out who I am, I'm more than happy to do that but as far as me seeking them, I've done my duty and I'm happy with that."

"I started the testing in August and the actual harvesting took place on January $2^{nd}$ of the following year. The process took several months, but to me it feels like it went by pretty fast. It was an outpatient procedure. My husband drove me in early that morning, I completed the process and we were finished by noon and I went home. That was on a Friday, and I was back at work that Monday. I never missed a day of work. I had complications from the actual procedure.

There was slight pain, but it was totally, definitely bearable. If I got a call again I wouldn't have any questions about doing it again. A lot of people are apprehensive though, when you say that there may be pain involved. But you're saving a life. I personally don't see the correlation between saving a life and pain. They say what does love have to do with it? Well I say what does pain have to do with it. You're possibly saving someone's life and wouldn't you want someone to do the same if you were in that predicament."

"I'm just blessed to have had the opportunity. I'm constantly trying to talk to other people but I find that, unfortunately, it's not of those things that that you can coax people into doing. And I'm not sure if you really want to whole heartedly coax them in, especially if you find out that they are a match and then they get to that point where they say no. Because to me, that's something hard to tell a person, 'we've found a match but they don't want to do it.' Even up until the week of the procedure I had the opportunity to say that I did not want to do it, and to me that would have been the worst thing. And it was funny because I even started driving a little more carefully because I didn't want to get into any accidents, I didn't want to do anything to jeopardize possibly saving someone's life. To me it's the closest thing to being an angel. I do think that we need to find a way to educate people more.

"When I was teaching, we were doing this unit on making a difference in someone's life. I always tell students the reason why I teach. I don't teach to make a living, I teach to make a difference. The year I became a donor I received all kinds of blessings. That was the year I became pregnant with my wonderful son.

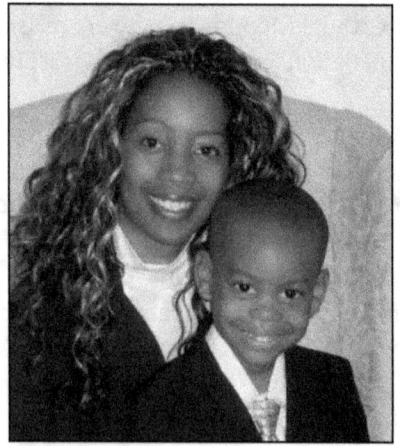

**Lummie Harris and son Jalen**

**Meet Kevin Allen** – He is a former football player, financial advisor and was a contestant on the Apprentice TV show.

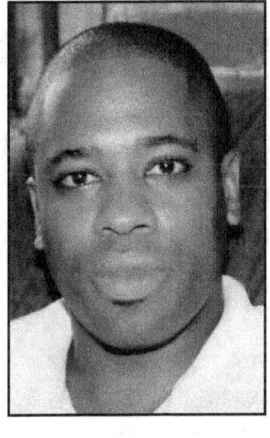 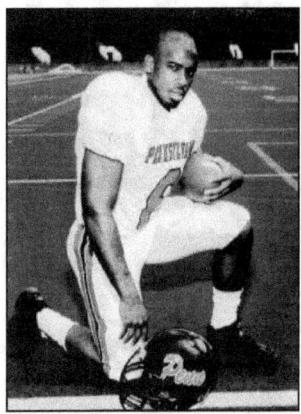

"I remember very vividly being the only Black person on the bus with my football team. We were responding to an appeal to become bone marrow donors. I recall I did not know anything about bone marrow donations."

" Some five years later while on a family vacation my younger brother Eric became ill. He was taken to the hospital, diagnosed and immediately admitted. He had leukemia. As it turned out, I was a perfect match for a donor transplant."

"Little did I realize, five years earlier, that I would be in position to help save a life – my brother's life."

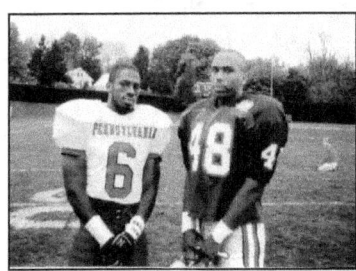

**Kevin and brother Eric**

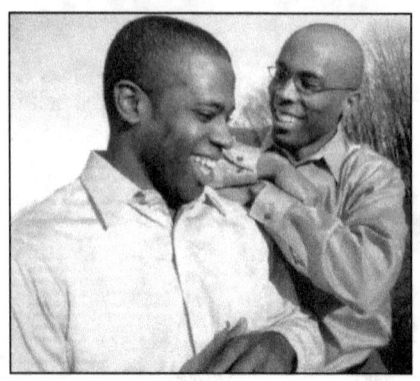

**Kevin and Eric**

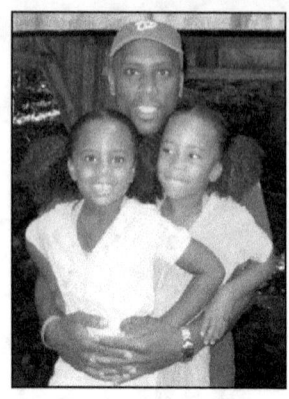

**Eric and his twin daughters**

"I would strongly urge anyone who has not registered, to make it a priority. With Blacks being underrepresented on the National Marrow Donor Registry, it is imperative that we step up and do what we have always done – help one another.

Note: Kevin's brother Eric is now the father of twin girls and Kevin the proud father of a new born.

In 2000 Cherie Fairfax was a frequent blood donor. She worked for the Red Cross and on one drive, she also signed up to be a marrow donor. It was seven years later, while working on a construction project she received a call from the National Marrow Donor Program. The caller identified herself and began to tell Cherie she was a potential match for someone. Cherie, in the midst of a very busy schedule, was hardly listening to the caller, believing it was some kind of sales call. Then the caller said the magic words that caught Cherie's attention, "You could save someone's life." At that moment Cherie recalls, "I dropped everything and began to listen. It had been five years since I signed up for the registry and I had completely forgotten. But those words, 'I could save a life', really reached home for me."

"I was told I was a match for a 38 year old gentleman with acute leukemia. I knew that whatever it would take, I was ready to step up to the plate to help save a life. I then went to the hospital for a series of tests and a complete physical to make sure there was no risk to me or the potential donor." While Cherie was tested, she discovered there were some irregularities with her white blood cells and she may not be able to be a donor. That's when I said, "Whatever it takes I want to go through with it. What do I need to do to build myself up to make sure I qualify?'

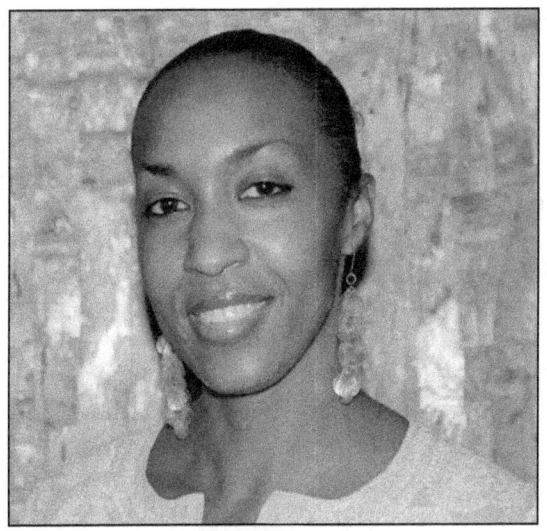

**Cherie Fairfax**

Cherie, determined to help save a life, was ready to meet the challenge. She was relieved when she discovered that she was able to be the donor. It was then she faced an unforeseen challenge. Friends and family began to question why she would put herself through all this for someone she didn't even know. "I was shocked and confused," she said, "As I listened to person after person, trying to discourage me from being a donor." "It was then I began to realize the fear and distrust many African

Americans have about doctors and the 'system', which they do not trust. I heard references to the Tuskegee Experiment and other incidents that brought about these concerns. That's when I had to let my friends and family, know that I was going to be a donor and hopefully save a life. I knew I would, because I believe that God put it in me, by choosing me to be this match. For me, the question stopped there."

"I realized that the patient, whom I have not yet met, was depending on me. I knew that if I backed out he may not live. I could only imagine the devastating effect it would have on him and his family if I said I changed my mind." Cherie had come face to face with a major decision and was confronted by many people who would dissuade her. Yet, Cherie felt a call from God to answer this request. When told you don't even know this man, she would reply, "Yes, you are right, but what if it was my son or daughter, or my father. Would I not want some stranger to be a donor?"

The doctors decided a stem cell transplant would work better for the donor. Cherie then began the routine to build her stem cells in preparation for the transplant. Doctors came to her home to give her shots to build her stem cell count. "The first three days went well. But on the fourth day, I did receive some discomfort, but kept in mind that my small discomfort was no match for the potential outcome should I not proceed. This is the time where some people drop out. I can only imagine the devastation for the patient and family to have their hopes suddenly dashed because someone wasn't willing to exchange some discomfort to save a life."

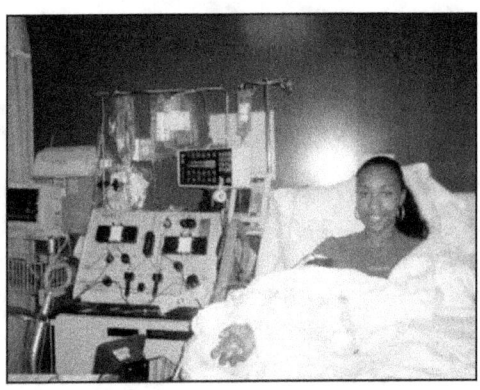

And then on June 22, 2007 Cherie entered Emory Hospital for the harvesting of her cells. At the same time, doctors were preparing the patient. It was then they discovered the patients white blood cells were somewhat compromised. The doctors began the treatment to build his white cell count so he would not reject the transplant. It was successful and he was prepared to receive the transplant. It was not known what city or state the patient was in. but whatever the case, all systems, were go.

On the following morning, Cherie received a call, that because the patient was a fairly large man, they needed more cells. "Without hesitation I returned and went through the process again. And I would do it all over again, if ever I am called."

After one year if both patient and donor agree, a meeting is scheduled. Cherie has not yet met the man for whom she donated, but hopes someday she will. Cherie advises, "Don't sign up if you think you will not go through with it if ever you are called. Don't just join the registry because it is a donor drive and your friends or co-workers are signing up. Because most matches are race specific, it is important that we, as African Americans, step up to the plate and do our part."

**Meet Adrein White, a** fourth grade student, and his mother Kim.

How does a fourth grade student respond to an assignment to name a hero? Does he look for an athlete or entertainer? Does he fantasize by thinking about what he would like to be? Or does he look closer to home? Andrein says he did not even take a second thought. He immediately knew who his hero was.

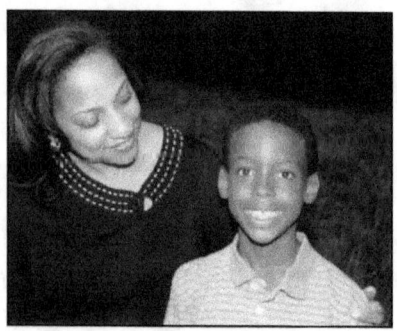

**Kim White and her son Adrein**

(Excerpts, from Adrien White's essay.)

"A hero is a person who saves people. My different hero is my mom, because she volunteered to help somebody she doesn't even know. " "Over nine years ago she gave a sample of blood to the National Marrow Donor Program. A few weeks ago they called and told her that you are a possible match for someone with Leukemia. Leukemia is a horrible disease of the blood. If my mom's blood is a match to the sick person then she will donate her bone marrow. A new bone marrow will make a person well."
"When the people called my mom, she said yes. Then dad said he was proud of her. That made her smile. I am proud of her too. Volunteering is a good thing to do."

Donors come from all walks of life, from a variety of ages and their motivation for becoming a donor varies. Tierra McClendon Is a student at Fort Valley State University in Fort Valley Georgia.

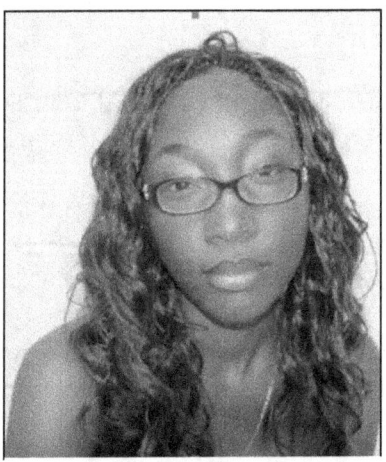

Tierra McClendon

"I signed up originally as a favor to my favorite teacher, Joanne Nobles, my Biology Instructor. I did not listen or fully understand just what I was signing up for but became fully aware of what I had done less than six months after I signed up. I understood the fact that it was for a great cause I didn't listen to what I was actually signing up for because of the fact that I didn't expect to be called at all. My teacher has been on the registry for 10 years and still has not been called."

"She just pulled me to the side one day in the student center, when they had a booth set up about marrow donation. She said, 'It'll only take five minutes.' She also said that she had been registered for ten years and hadn't been called. So I signed up and I wasn't even on the list for six months before they called me and said that I was a match."

I feel that it was a blessing for me as well as the patient because I actually had the opportunity to save another person's life who was only 20 years old- A year older than me. He has a whole life to live ahead of him and I'm honored to be able to assist him in fighting for that life."

Stacy Toney, Recruiter for the national Marrow Donor Program accompanied Tierra to EMORY Hospital for the procedure.

Tierra is a match for a 20 year old male not living in the United States. "I just pray that his body doesn't reject it and all goes well for the patient."

Tierra's mother is on the National Kidney Donor list, hoping to find a match. Her father is soon to be deployed to Iraq for the fourth tour of duty.

At the age of 19, Tierra has helped save a life.

# THE
# PATIENCE OF
# THE PATIENTS

Every day in hospital beds around the world people are facing life-threatening diseases. There is no level playing field. Unfortunately, race, color, and finance play a major role in who gets treated and how. While there are some things that will take time to correct, there is at least one thing we as Blacks can do other than just complain.

The numbers on the registry are low when it comes to Black participation. While there may be many reasons, I prefer to deal with the solutions. We must step up our educational awareness campaigns and reach more people with the message that we are our brother's and sister's keeper.

Many donor drives are motivated by someone known to a particular group of people in a workplace or church. Perhaps one of the things which must continually be stressed is that if you sign up to become a marrow donor because of a drive for someone you know, you should also consider that you may be a match for someone else. If, for any reason you change your mind after you are on the registry, please contact the proper registry and have your name removed,

For many patients they are told that they have found one or even several matches. The patient and their family have received a new ray of hope. However, too often the prospective donor cannot be reached or they have changed their mind. What a tragic let down. What a discouraging way to have ones hopes dashed because the donor backed out. If you move, please notify the registry. If you change your mind, let them know that you wish to be removed from the registry. You will be removed with NO questions asked.

According to the National Marrow Donor Program, more than 6,000 people are searching the registry for a match on any given day.

Finding a match for a patient who is Black is a challenge. Perhaps no one knows more about the disparities in patient care regarding transplants, than people like Cheryl Christian. Cheryl is the Bone Marrow Transplant Nurse Navigator for EMORY Hospital's Winship Cancer Institute.

For the past several years, Cheryl has been searching registries worldwide trying to find donors for patients with leukemia and other blood borne diseases. Her responsibility is to coordinate care and negotiate patients through transplants. When Cheryl sits down at her computer to begin her search she is well aware that the results of her search are directly related to the race of the patient.

Cheryl Christian, RN

"I have sat at my computer to search for a matching marrow donor for a white patient and pulled up hundreds and sometime thousands of potential matching donors. And there are times I sit at this same computer with the sane resources available, but if the patient is Black or African American, the results will be dramatically different. I may find as little as none and in some instances I may find ten possible matching donors. This is very discouraging. And to compound this, in so many cases when we reach out to the prospective donor, they cannot be located or in some tragic cases, they have changed their mind and no longer want to be considered a donor."

Again, this further emphasizes the need for proper training and information during donor drives to assure that the person joining the registry is fully aware that the need may arise for them to become a donor. In some cases the person has be motivated to sign up because they have a friend, co-worker or family member who needs a transplant. Once the drive is over, and the person for whom they registered to help, has either found a match or has been unsuccessful and has expired, they sometime lose interest.

This also reinforces the need to make sure you provide adequate information regarding how to contact you and notify the registry if you change your address. It is perhaps equally important that if for any reason you change your mind, it is imperative that you notify the registry to have your name removed. Your name will be removed – no questions asked.

Cheryl recalls some of her most discouraging and encouraging moments. "It is very sad to know that you could have helped someone live or have a better life and you cannot find a matching donor. Because the pool from which we draw to find donors has so few Blacks registered, it is very difficult finding a donor that can help save a life. We have the treatment, but need the donors. But it is rewarding to see a patient receive a transplant and go on to live a better life after the transplant. I recall one of my happiest moments was when a 19 year old female had leukemia and her sister was a perfect match. But somehow after the transplant she relapsed. We were able to find several unrelated donors. She had another transplant but was not expected to live. We did not think she would make it out of the hospital. Today, she is very much alive, has finished college and travels extensively. That is what makes this position rewarding."

**Meet Sonya Jones,** former postal worker. Sonya is married with two children.

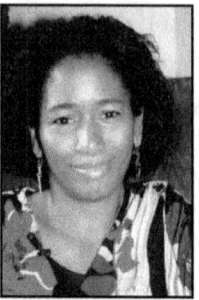

"I have chronic monogynies leukemia. I found out October 2001. I had a bruise on my leg that would never go away."

Sonya had several visits to see a doctor, and then the news.

"At that time, I didn't know what leukemia was I thought it was a cold that would disappear. Finally had a follow up appointment with the doctor and was told I had leukemia. I was totally devastated, because I was told I had cancer... of the blood. My first reaction was I'm going to die."

"At first, it was painful. I would have bad migraines, would ball up in a knot for hours from stomach aches and my bones being weak. I had small children and didn't want them to see me that way, but I had no choice. The pain was excruciating."

"When I was waiting for a match they found several, but they all changed their mind. I was devastated. By the grace of God I no longer need a match."

"The only way I have survived is because I found God. I am now in remission."

**Meet Deidre C. Hudson,** survivor.

"First and foremost I give all the praise and glory to my Lord and Savior God Almighty Jesus Christ!! I am 28 years old. On January 7, 2006 I was given a terminal diagnosis of Acute Myelogenous Leukemia (AML) Cancer of the blood. I was transferred to a hospital that was four hours away from my home for a period of nine months. The doctors told my family that if I made it to the next morning it would be a miracle. They said call all of the family together."

"I was on life-support system for seven days because I had pneumonia in one lung and it was difficult to breathe. My kidneys failed, and I was placed on a dialysis machine for almost three months. I received six rounds of chemotherapy treatments. I had a stem cell collection performed. I was scheduled to have a bone marrow transplant, but didn't have a match. But God has worked things out for me."

"I was made over. I had to learn how to walk, feed, and dress myself all over again. I am now off the dialysis machine; my kidneys are working normally. During all of that, I was five months pregnant. I miscarried while on life support the day after I started my first chemotherapy treatment. My baby girl, Makayla Andrea, is now resting and watching over me in heaven as "My Angel.""

"I said all of that to say you're now looking at a blessed and anointed child of God!! Free of cancerous blood cells!! Now, I'm looking forward to the many more blessings that God has in store for me. I know he didn't do all of this for me to not find my purpose driven life!! I know if he did it for me he will do it for YOU. You must trust and believe that all things are possible, when God is placed first!!"

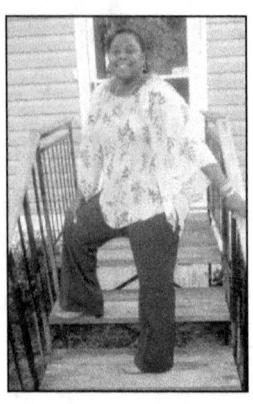

**Deidre C. Hudson**

"I'm just too blessed to be stressed and too anointed to be disappointed. I have experienced that whatever God brings you to he will bring you all the way through. I leave you with this: be kinder than necessary, for everyone you meet is fighting some kind of battle. I plan to live well, laugh often, and love with all my heart, while giving praise to God. So if you didn't get anything else out of my message...know that everything happens for a reason in every season. Hold your head high in the sky!! Through all of this I am still smiling. I've returned back to work. Mentally and physically I'm healed!! Don't get caught up and miss your blessings. Get busy living, because God is true to His word. A special thanks to my husband Mandell and my family and friends for hanging in there with me through this trying time of my life. One friend in particular, Avis, who initially made me go back to the hospital one more time. The doctors said if I had waited another day there would have been nothing they could do for me."

**Meet Taylor John -** fourteen year old high school student.

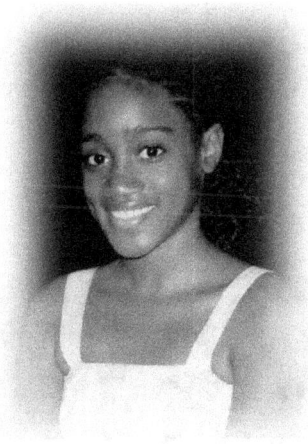

"I'm in 10<sup>th</sup> grade, and when I grow up I want to be a hematologist. My favorite subject is science. I got an A in science and I will graduate in 2012. I'm going to college. I want to go to Emory, to be a hematologist. I got my mind made up."

Wislene John is Taylor's mother. She has been an educator for twelve years. She speaks passionately about her daughter. "Taylor was diagnosed with sickle cell shortly after birth, so we've lived with the disease for about for almost fifteen years. So we've traveled the road with the illness, in and out of the hospital, with multiple blood transfusions. I stopped counting after the thirtieth hospitalization so she's been in the hospital probably about 50 to 60 times. Sometimes she was hospitalized for three or four days and other times up to two weeks. The beginning part of 2008 was the worst part of Taylor's life. She had a really, really serious bout with the disease, and had multiple complications. But prior to that, back in 2005 we did check the registry and she didn't have a match. She was tested to be typed and they ran it through the system and there wasn't a match. And then about a year ago, I was told that there was a match in the registry for cord blood, but the size of the cord was too small. So they wouldn't risk starting the procedure in case they needed to go back and draw some more cells from the cord they wouldn't be able to. So they need to have a live person that they could go back and extract more stem cells and redo the transplant if need be,. So we decided to start a campaign because we believe that there is someone somewhere that is a match."

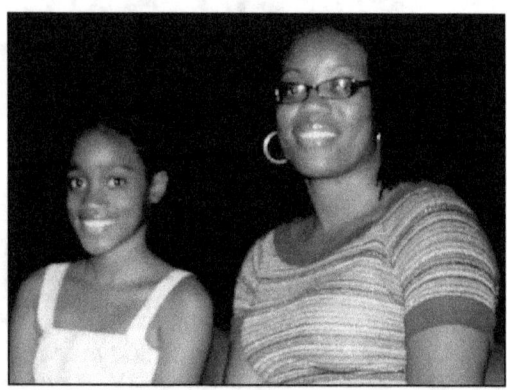

**Taylor John and her mother Wislene**

"Things happen in mysterious ways and God orchestrates it. I was in the mall one Saturday and my pastor called me from Virginia, and said 'Wislene, have you ever thought about a bone marrow transplant for Taylor?' She had been in the hospital for several weeks prior, and I said 'yes I have but, you know, there isn't a match?' And he said 'why don't you call them, (the National Marrow donor Program) we can do something through the church. I said okay and called Egleston a few days later. The young lady at Egleston, said 'well actually the representative from the National Marrow Donor Program (NMDP) just called me looking for a family that would be willing to be featured.' My response was 'wow, perfect timing'.

"So, Stacy Toney, representative from NMDP, and I, got in touch. She asked if she could come that Sunday.  Stacy came to my church to basically educate the congregation. She spoke before all three services, which was probably over 3,000 people. She returned two weeks later and we had over two hundred donors register that day. So we continued our journey, and went on radio station WAOK 1380 with Derrick Boazman He, was so moved, that he pledged to help us get 1400 people on the registry."

"Taylor expresses herself so eloquently stating, "I feel thankful that so many people would love to help me, and I'm hoping for one of those people to be a match to save my life; and not just my life but many others. Just because I'm the only face that you see, doesn't mean that I'm the only person that you're helping. You can be a match for any other person out there. You're just signing up with me but you don't have to be my match. That's what I love about this, - it's not just about me. It's about everyone."

"I'll be fifteen on my birthday, August 15th. I like dancing. I used to dance with my church, but then my illness came back, so I haven't danced in a while. I like going to sickle cell camp. That is something I really do enjoy. I like spending time with my family down in Florida, and I just like hanging out sometimes going to see movies and being a normal teenager. "

"Really I don't go a lot of places, I mostly stay at home but when I do go out I either go to the mall or go see a movie with my family. My favorite singing group is Mary Mary. I like the song God In Me."

## Deborah Price shares her Unrequested Journey

*And we know that all things work together for good to them that love God, and to them who are the called according to His purpose. Rom. 8:28*

The dream of most women is to become a mother someday, and to be the sports mom, dance mom, Girl Scout, Cub Scout den mother. For most it is a dream come true coupled with fears, laughter and lots of anxieties.

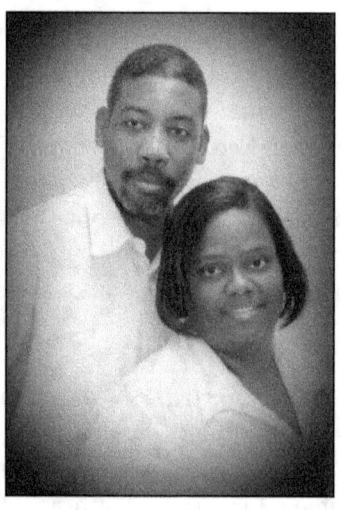

Vincent & Delores Price

December 1995 after being diagnosed with pneumonia I was congratulated on a long awaited pregnancy. What a wonderful announcement. How thrilled we were to know, that God trusted us enough to allow us the opportunity to be guardians of one of His most precious gifts; a child. January 4, 1996 I returned to my Ob-GYN for a checkup and ultrasound. To our surprise we not only were having a baby but instead we were having triplets. After nine months of pregnancy I gave birth to three healthy baby boys.

Once we came home we settled in and an unexpected telephone call came two weeks later. The joy and excitement of new babies was soon replaced with tears and great fear. The MD health department called to say that my baby Nile was diagnosed with Sickle Cell disease SS. My heart sank as the nurse was giving me information for the Hematology/Oncology clinic at Johns Hopkins. We went for our initial appointment only to leave before the checkup began. The doctor asked my husband and I what was Sickle Cell. I knew this was not the place for my baby. We were referred to Children's National Hospital and that wasn't any better. At exactly thirteen months old Nile had his first pain crisis. He experienced the hand foot syndrome in which he swelled so badly. This began the first of many long hospital admissions.

By age five Nile had had about 60 to 100 hospital admissions. He had suffered many painful crisis, bone necrosis and pneumonias. We did all we knew to make sure he had as normal a life as his brothers did. He has played sports but with limitations. He has lots of limitations on his life for the past 13 years. His pediatrician was the one to give him the best care because of her knowledge of Sickle Cell. She discovered that his really bad sinus was the cause of many of his crisis. She began to manage his sinus problems and we saw a decrease in the number of crisis and hospitalizations.

In February 2002 our family relocated to Richmond, VA. We

were referred to the Hemoc clinic at VCU Health systems where things began to look up for my son. Nile was seen by the best in the area. He was not as sick as before and he actually was able to do more activities and  spend time away from home. In March 2005 Nile started getting really sick again and this time we had the big scare. Nile suffered from an acute chest syndrome. This is a type of pneumonia that can be severely devastating to Sicklers. After a week in the PICU and having an exchange transfusion, he was well enough to come out to the floor and later go home. The Hemoc team later discussed with us the need to try Hydroxy Urea. This is a very old chemo drug that was discovered to work wonders on people with sickle cell disease. It sort of tricks the body into making fetal hemoglobin. Fetal hemoglobin does not sickle so this is why it is sort of considered to be a miracle drug. At least it did for a while. For three and a half years Nile was just as healthy and normal as his brothers. In 2008 he began to start having pain crisis again. By the fall Nile had become a frequent flyer at the hospital. Everyone there knew him and the family personally. He suffered yet more pneumonia and everyday was a day of living with pain. He returned to the hospital after Christmas and every other week after that we were living there. They were not able to control his pain unless several narcotics were onboard. By the end of January he was taken out of school because he was just too sick to return. By February he was now living in the hospital. His hematologist pulled us into consult to say that he needed a bone marrow transplant because his condition was really getting worse. She feared he would suffer a stroke or other organ damage. All of which is not reversible. We agreed but of course with many reservations and lots of fear.

At the end of February the other two boys were tested to see if they were a donor match for Nile. We all were so hopeful and the boys were excited to possibly be a match for their brother. The idea of Nile being cured of this dreadful disease was the best news we had in a very long time. The transplant coordinator called two weeks later to say the brothers were not a match. This was a devastating blow. And as you may not expect, parents are rarely a match themselves. We weren't. The coordinator said the search would now go to the national bone marrow registry. She informed us that it could take awhile because of the low number of African Americans on the registry. The national Bone Marrow registry has approximately 7 million registered donors and of this number only 600,000 are African Americans. As the search began we too began to do our part to educate and get people registered. Our son along with thousands of others was in need of the lifesaving transplant. The first weekend in March was one of four Donor drives that we and our friends began. Sadly to say, at each drive the turn out to register was incredible but they all consisted of other races readily agreeing to register to possibly be of help to save my son's life. The drive that was the greatest disappointment was the weekend that the Pittsburgh Steelers were in town for a charity event. Our friends were there to do a drive and there were so many people. We had over 80 people to register that day. The disappointment was the fact that only 4 of those people were African American and only two football players registered and my child was there talking to countless people. Hundreds of people there to see the child who was in desperate need of this life saving transplant and only the people of other races were moved with enough compassion to help. While grateful as we were for them joining the registry, unfortunately they would not be a good match for

Nile. We needed and African American donor and we needed them soon.

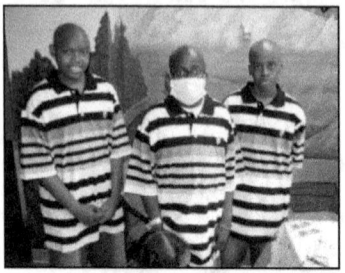

Jordan, Nile, Immanuel

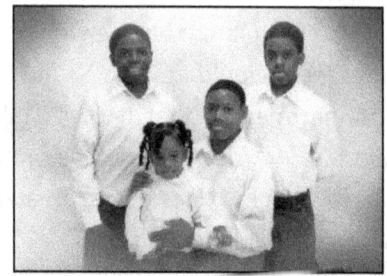

Nile, Olivia, Jordan, Immanuel

Thank God for answering prayers. By the middle of May the BMT coordinator called with great news. From the National Registry two perfect matched donors had been found. While being a matched donor you still have the opportunity to say no. Thankfully the donors were in agreement. The first donor was tested and she agreed to continue with the donation of her bone marrow. On July 21$^{st}$ Nile received his new stem cells and by the end of August he was 100% donor cells and Sickle cell disease free.

If it had not been for this wonderful woman, my son would still be battling this horrific disease and I would still be wondering if I'll get to see him graduate from college or get married. Today, thanks to a donor, we are planning his future and enjoying hearing him talk about his plans for becoming a Senator. We did not request to take this journey but since we had to go through this I thank God for the person who decided one day to give the gift of life to another person. Our prayer is that other African Americans would give the gift of life by becoming a registered bone marrow donor before it is too late.

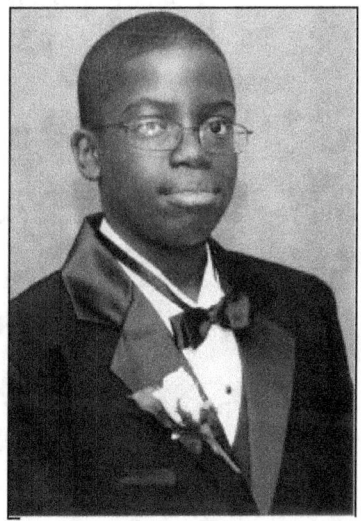

Nile Price

Deborah Lundy tells her story. "My son Chris was diagnosed with sickle when he was two months old. We took him to the doctor on other occasions but he was originally misdiagnosed. We didn't know much about sickle cell but we knew it was serious enough for us to take him to Atlanta from our home in Rome, Georgia, where he could be treated. For the next several years Chris had several crises. This would happen about once a year, which pales in comparison to others with the disease. By the time he reached 9th grade it became more serious and the crises became more frequent."

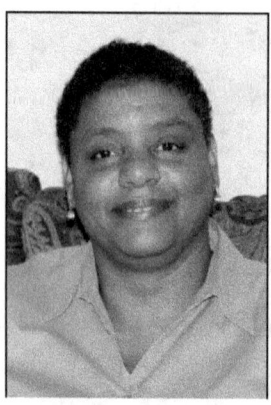

**Deborah Lundy**

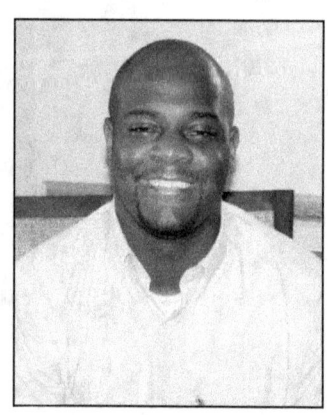

**Chris Lundy**

Chris is now twenty two and is a Student Services Specialist at Georgia Highlands College. He reflects on those days as though it was yesterday. "I remember very vividly", he recalls, "being in and out of the hospital and having several operations. I had my spleen removed when I was two and had gall bladder surgery at the age of five, It wasn't easy. By the fall of 1999 while in the 10th grade things began to get worse."

"The doctors suggested a marrow transplant. I was nervous about the idea having been through surgery before, I knew it would set me back in school and I would have to leave my friends in Rome Georgia and travel to Atlanta for the treatment. But we have a very close and supportive family and I knew that they were with me. My family planned several donor drives and the doctors at Children's health care of Atlanta suggested we test my younger brother who was ten years old. The test would have to be a six point match for the marrow transplant to work. My brother was a perfect six."

Chris' brother Warren would then be called upon to possibly save his brother's life. Warren recalls his reaction. "I was really for it. There was no hesitation. It's my brother. Let's get on with it. We have a strong family and we always stick together. I don't like hospitals so my thought was let me get in, get this done and get out of there. We went in about six am and by 2 PM it was all over and they wanted me to stay overnight. My thought was, no, let me get out of here and go home. I was ready to go. I did my part. We left and headed home."

For Chris it was a tremendous blessing and he says he is forever grateful for his brother for saving his life. He also expresses his gratitude to Children's Health Care of Atlanta. (CHOA) for the service they provided. Chris states with deep emotion, "The doctors at CHOA were always very concerned and cautious during the entire time. They did not take any short cuts. After surgery I had a brief battle with Graff Host disease but it was only a temporary set- back. I was on mediation from 7 am to 1 PM and then again 7 PM to 1am."

"On January 17, 2001, I recall as though it was yesterday, I had an experience I will never forget. I was at a basketball game and felt my head itching. I went to scratch my head and then could not take my arm down. I fell forward, face down on a concrete pavement. I ended up in Egleston Hospital. I have not had any problems since that day."

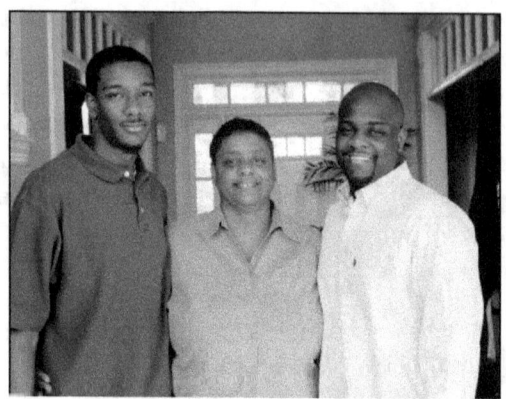

**Warren Deborah and Chris Lundy**

Warren who is now much taller than his brother Chris says he would do it all over again if needed. "I only have one brother and I am grateful and humble about what I did. I needed a brother to look up to and go to for advice. I have that brother."

Akim DeShay expresses his gratitude for being alive. "I was married, 32 and did not have an active lifestyle. I smoked cigarettes and drank beer and liquor every weekend. I did not attend church. I spent my Sunday's recuperating from Saturday nights. My wife was pregnant with our second child at the time."

"It was sometime in autumn in 2003. I noticed the shortness of breath after climbing one flight of stairs. Then came the night sweats. From time to time I experienced blurry vision. Then my throat started to swell. My Lymph nodes were tender and big. "

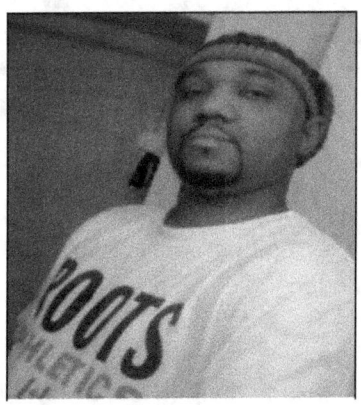

**Akim DeShay**

"I was diagnosed with Mono by one doctor - A throat infection by another doctor and a 'perfect' case of tonsillitis by an ear nose and throat specialist."

"It was getting close to Thanksgiving now. As it got closer to that day I got worse. I was feeling flu-like symptoms - Unusual weakness, headaches, sweating, Feeling very hot, loss of appetite and even some dizziness."

"Thanksgiving came and I didn't eat a thing. I never left the bed. I laid in bed Friday and Saturday with the worst stomach ache I had ever had in my life. My wife had enough. She called my mother. My mother said, "Akiim, if you are not sure about your relationship with Jesus then you need to go to the hospital." I thought she was just talking but she said it again. And this time she made herself clear, as if it had been decided. All I could say was "OK, Ill go" We went to the local hospitals ER.

**The Shock....**

"So there I sat awaiting this "bad" news. What's the worst it could be? - A very bad ulcer? Then she came, a young female doctor. She told me she was going to be straight forward." "According to my blood tests there was a 95% chance I had Leukemia."

"I was in shock. I really didn't even know what Leukemia was. The only time I ever heard it before I was in Junior High. The lady down the street suddenly died of it. She was 33. I am 32. "I'm gonna die". Tears started streaming."

"Then the doctor said something I NEVER thought I would hear from a doctor. She asked "Are You Christians? Would you like me to pray?" I said yes. Little did I know God was already stepping in. I thought doctors were all Atheists, but here she was leading us in prayer in open in the ER in front of the nurses and all. I don't even remember what she said, not a word. As it turned out she didn't even work there. She was helping out that day because her sister was admitted with something life threatening and they were so busy so she volunteered. That was the only day she worked there. She even came to visit me when I was getting my chemo in a different hospital. She is now my family doctor."

"I was so terrified I could not cry right, Just tears. I worried about my wife and kids. What's going to happen to them if I die? My wife will be a single mother. My kids will never know their father."

"Who will pay the bills? I had no more vacation time and my decision to wait until age 35 to get disability and life insurance has left my family in a bind. I felt so guilty and helpless. I was in a position where I had no control of my life. I had no way to make sure my family had a place to live. Will they get evicted? Will they have to leave town. I was powerless. The tears were coming hard. I was frantic but quite."

"I called to the house and asked to speak to my father-in-law. He is a Missionary Baptist Reverend in MS. He came to see me. I told him how I felt. I also told him that I was ashamed for not preparing my family for the worst and most of all too shamed to call on God. This is because I had not had a close relationship with God in a long time and it seemed insulting to only call on him when I'm sick. I felt like I did not deserve his help. My father in-law talked to my about the book of Job. How God allowed the devil to do horrible things to Job and his family and how God rewarded Job because his faith in Him never faltered."

"But the most important thing I remember, He said "if you believe that Jesus is real, just the same way you believe that floor exists under your bed, you will be healed and God will take your fear from you and hold on to it." Something happened then. It was kind of a blur, but I remember feeling kind of strange. I remember saying that I do believe that Jesus is real. I remember thinking about the floor and how Jesus, who I can't see, is just is as real as that floor that I can see. He said a prayer, then left. That's when I noticed my tears were gone. I felt a big sense of relief. I felt that my family was going to be safe and that I have the power to fight this illness and beat it. It was as if God touched me and took my fears away."

"I prayed that god would take care of my family while I was gone. And then it started happening. Soon after my last paycheck was deposited in my account the phone calls began.... from Friends, coworkers, relatives, friends of relatives. Although we did not even talk to anyone about our situation, everyone who called said they were sending money."

"He gave my wife strength beyond belief. Although she was 5 months pregnant, had our 4yr old daughter diagnosed with autism, and a husband who was in the hospital she was able to take over and do what had to be done. She made all the phone calls and waited in long lines for Social Security, Food Stamps, Rental assistance, medical assistance, and everything else we needed. She prayed and encouraged everyone who called about us. You have unbelievable strength baby and I love you."

**The Miracles....**

"Cancer treatment is what they say it is, "Pain and Suffering" - A lot. But with the God on your side you can stand strong. I spent Christmas and New Years in that hospital bed."

"That's when the news got worse."

"Although the Oncologist predicted I had an 80% chance of going into remission, the chemo only killed half of the Leukemia cells. My prognosis dropped. At this time I was much more likely to die than live. My only chance of survival was a Bone Marrow Transplant."

"She referred me to another doctor who I call my bone marrow doctor. He told me he thought I had a 40% chance based on my age and current health as long as they could find a donor. (I later found out that my prognosis was more like 10-12%) Then the bad news, I have one sibling, my sister, and there was only a 25%

chance of her being a match. If not, I had a 40% chance of finding a donor in the National Donors registry because I'm black. Whites had a 95% chance."

"I went through two more rounds of Chemo. Two weeks into the third treatment the Lord answered our prayers again. I got a call from my wife. 'She's a perfect match!' My sister and only sibling was a perfect match for my transplant."

"I underwent a high dose regiment of Chemo to kill all of my bone marrow and then after a week received the transplant on Good Friday of all days. Three weeks later I was released with a successful transplant. That was in 2004. I still have issues related to the transplant and it is not easy from day to day. But I am here and have the opportunity to raise my kids."

**MORE....**

"A year after my transplant one of my best friends from Rochester who had joined the donor registry became a match for an 18yr old from the Bronx. He was that youngster's only chance. And in 2006 months ago I got an opportunity to meet him, shake his hand, and talk about college."

"Good thing he is a forgiving God - Because I never gave anything in my life to help others. I remember when the Blood donation truck would come up to the job. I was like "not me". You know how we get. We don't trust anybody especially with a needle. I say it's a good thing that he is a forgiving God because during my treatment I received blood transfusions more than 20 times to help keep me alive even though I never gave anything. But through the grace of God I was able to receive. There were 20 people who I never met, who gave. I owe them."

www.blackbonemarrow.com

While attending a Sickle Cell Conference here in Atlanta I met several patients and their families. One of the people I met was a young lady who was beaming with joy. Her name was Aaron Washington. I then met her mother Joyce. Joyce shares Aaron's Story.

"My name is Joyce Washington, Aaron's mom. Aaron has 3 sibling, Tayla, the oldest, Maya, the middle child, and Jeremiah her baby brother. Aaron is the youngest of the sisters. Aaron's Father and I were high school sweet hearts; college educated and began our beautiful family. I was a stay at home mom, managing the household and the unexpected chronic illness that Aaron suffered from. I can only assume that the financial as well as the emotional strain on our family, my ex-husband must have felt was the reason he let our family after a 11yr marriage and 17yr relationship. "

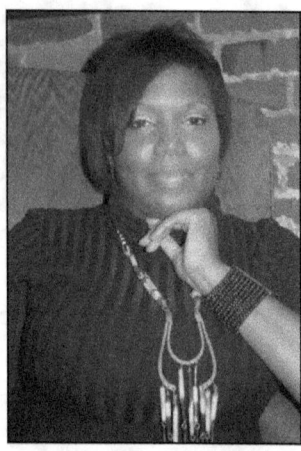

Joyce Washington

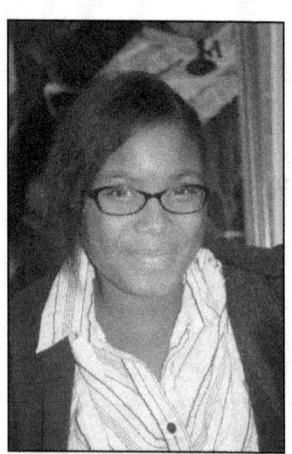

Aaron Washington

"Now a divorced single mom, dealing with the sole responsibility of raising 4 children and Aaron with a chronic illness, it was very hard. I had to struggle to find and keep a job that would allow me time off if and when Aaron got sick. After job after job, I felt the only way I can support my family and work around the many doctor's appointments, not just Aaron's, but also the rest of my children's, I would have to start my own home base business. And that is just what I did. And so our story goes:"

"Aaron had severe sickle cell disease. By age 11, she had endured Acute Chest Syndrome, 3 strokes with therapy for recovery, chronic blood transfusions every 3 to 4 weeks, treatment for iron overload, meningitis, countless hospitalization and doctors and clinic visits."

"After she experienced her 2nd stroke while on transfusions, which was needed to prevent her from having strokes, the doctors could not assure us that the transfusion therapy could prevent Aaron from having life threatening and debilitating strokes that may lead to her death."

"As her mother, I always thought about Aaron's quality of life, and how long could she live like that? "

"At that point the doctors told us about BMT (Bone Marrow Transplant) for sickle cell. A perfect sibling match would be the protocol for consideration. We were all tested for a perfect HLA, her 2 sisters Tayla and Maya, her brother, Jeremiah, and her father and I. The test came back, NO MATCH! I prayed that God would make a way."

"Weeks later while at one of Aaron routine blood transfusions, and check up, Aaron's doctors asked if we would volunteer to consider participating in a research study for severe sickle cell."
"This study is to try a new treatment for sickle cell using bone

morrow transplantation from a close non-matched sibling. We were told, in order for successful BMT treatment for Sickle cell the donor and host has to be a 6 out of 6 perfect match. Aaron and her oldest sister, Tayla wad a 5 out of 6 match, closes enough to be part of the study. Prayers answered! Hope at last!"

"Aaron was told about the risks and it would not be easy. They told her about the side effects from the chemo that will kill her bone marrow to replace it with her sisters. She was told how it will make her sick and not feel so good and how all her long beautiful hair will fall out, how she can develop GVHD (Graft Versus Host Disease) and maybe rejection, worst case, she may die. Aaron thought a little about it, and said, "I have been in pain all my life, and lots of needles, going back and forth to the hospital, feeling sick all the time, and about my hair, it will grow back. I have no hope with sickle cell, but with God and this BMT I may have a chance". Then she turned to me and said "mommy I want to do it". I said, ok, and we never looked back."

"So our journey begins and with any journey comes challenges and set- backs. After Aaron had her 2$^{nd}$ stroke we had to wait a year from stroke before we could start the BMT process. We were getting close 3 more months from January and she would have been one year passed stroke when she experienced her yet 3$^{rd}$ stroke. With this stroke she could not talk or move the right side of her body. She regained most of what she lost, and we had to begin again."

"With a year to prepare mentally and financially for the BMT we began to put a support team around us and save funds for when we had to go into the long hospital stay for transplant. I worked hard building my fitness company Fit 1 Fitness. We made plans for my other 3 children; it seemed overwhelming as a single mother when the unspeakable happened. The landlord decided not to pay the mortgage on the home that we were renting, and

It went into foreclosure. The home was also full of mold and would not be good for Aaron to come out of BMT back home. So with the help of our wonderful friends, neighbors and support team and a new home, we once again regained most of what we lost and we began again."

"Sunday March 23$^{rd}$, check in day at Children's Hospital at Egleston."

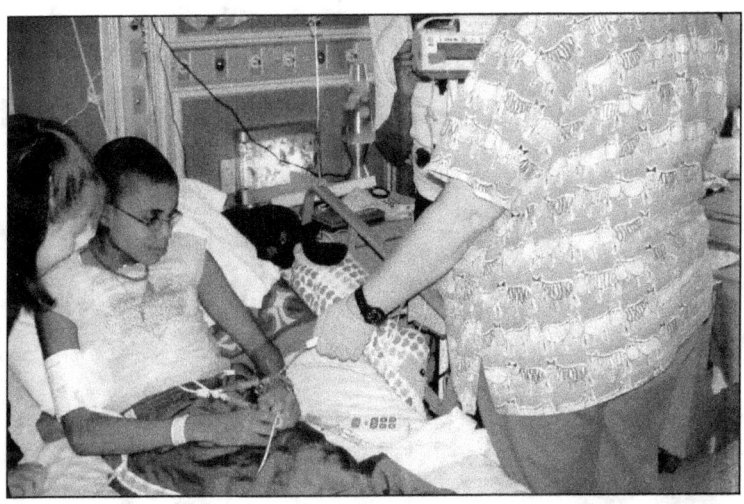

"Because of the high doses of chemo that Aaron would be receiving, with the thought of her hair just falling out, Aaron decided to take control and have her head saved by her father on the day she checked into the Children's hospital at Egleston. Aaron's Dad with some of his co-workers and friends shaved their head in support of Aaron."

"She had the most perfect head. Her big angle eye's just beamed through. She was the most beautiful bald headed person I have ever seen."

"We went in with hope, faith and trust in God! Aaron just shined with hope in her heart. She went into surgery to have her central line put in and her own marrow harvested. "

"Her big sister Tayla checked in on April 3rd for her marrow harvest to give to her sister. Tayla did not think twice about what she was giving up. She said she would do anything to make her baby sister well. Tayla does not see her gift as a sacrifice. To her, it was something she had to do."

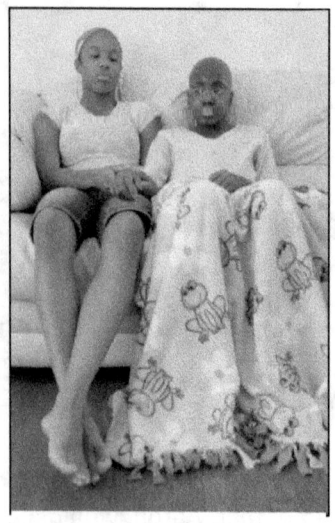
Tayla and Aaron

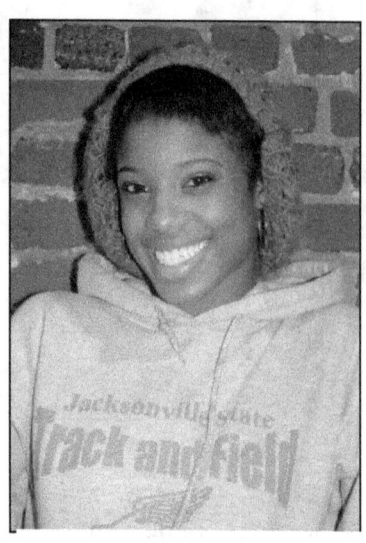
Tayla Washington

"April 5th, we call it, Aaron's rebirth, the day she received her sister's marrow. She received her new life and new beginning without sickle cell disease."

"Aaron did everything the doctors and nurses asked of her with no complaints. She made friends with everyone, from the kitchen to the cleaning staff at the hospital. Aaron and I would get up early in the morning to do her laps around the nurses station even when she felt bad. She greeted everyone who came into her room with a big smile and a hello. She went through her pain and sickness with such grace and dignity."

"Weeks pass as we receive the news that her sister's marrow is holding on and she is now 100% donor and sickle cell free. It has been 12 weeks since we began the journey of going home. With each day, bills were piling up and work was being lost. My fitness business remained unmanaged and that was my hope to recover financial loss."

"With everything our family was facing, the last thing our family needed to worry about is food to eat, keep our utilities on and paying rent. It was hard to come up with funds to put gas in our car to get Aaron back and forth to the clinic."

"Her recovery was proceeding when, on June 19, Aaron was rushed to the hospital after her brother Jeremiah found her having a seizure. The doctors determined she suffered a stroke. They also found a problem with her colon that could have led to a deadly infection, the greatest post-transplant risk. "

"Surgery was successful, Doctors had to remove half of her colon due to GVHD and they had to perform an eilostomy. Damage from the stroke appears minimal. Complication from the Stoma ostomy has been causing added problems."

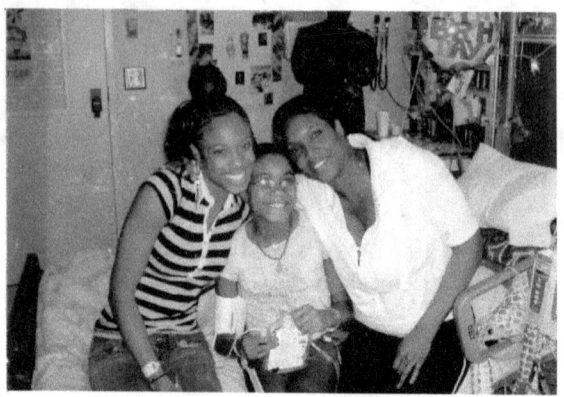

Maya, Aaron and Joyce

"September thru October, Aaron has been hospitalized for staph infections, bacterial infections in her blood stream, pneumonia and malnutrition. She is on continuous IV med and fluids to maintain her blood level and that in its self is hard on her body. Even though Aaron is 190 days post transplant she still needs the same amount of meds and care as she did on day 1 of transplant. Doctors hope that with Aaron's surgery of reversing her ostomy, her body can begin to heal again."

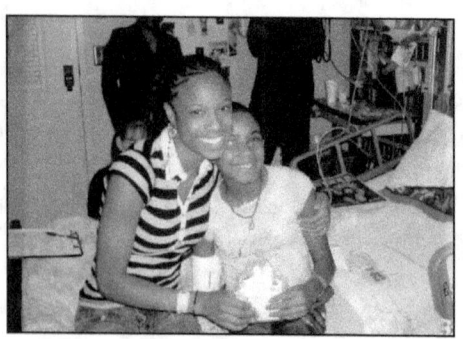
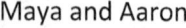

Maya and Aaron

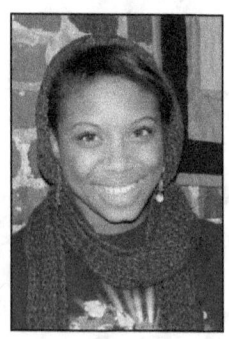

Maya

"Aaron's sisters, Maya and Tayla talk candidly about their

experiences growing up. They recall with humor the many days they spent protecting their little sister. They defended her with fierce passive tenacity to let others know about her illness. They reflect on the times they had to help her change her fluid bag in what they describe as "it sucked." Yet they both smile and say without hesitation, "we'd do it all over again if we had to."

"Aaron's most recent challenges have posed additional complications to her BMT. She needs more assistants for care that is not covered by our insurance, and I need to be able to recover household expenses and necessities. Our household income consists of child support which covers our rent, and Aaron's SSI. Because we are behind on everything we are left with nothing on which to survive. "

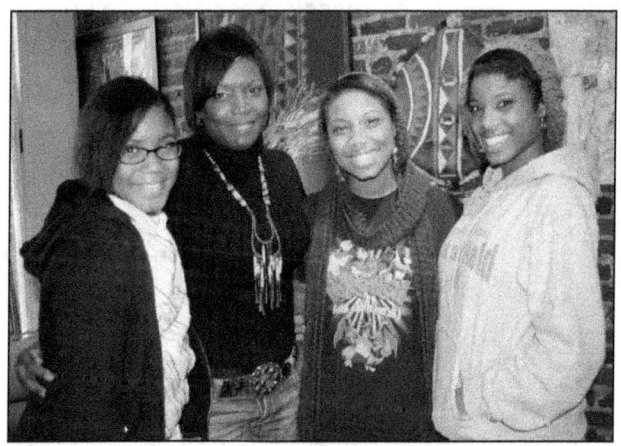

Aaron, Joyce, Maya and Tayla

"Our hope is that Aaron's spirit stays strong. This has been a long recovery for her and she still has a ways to go. Keep praying for us. And don't forget this little girl with the determination to live to give back to others. We welcome your support."

In September 2006: Suzanne Gordon and Joyce Washington

were strangers - brought together by a common, yet silent disease.

Suzanne Gordon is a mother of 4, two of whom suffer with Sickle Cell Disease. By age 3, her son Jaelin had been hospitalized through several episodes of Acute Chest Syndrome and many pain crises, he then began chronic transfusion therapy, which provided some relief from the effects of this illness. Nearly two years later, instead of transfusions, he was started on a medication which continued this relief. However, at age six, Jaelin spent 3 weeks in ICU on a ventilator and 3 more weeks in rehabilitation. For Suzanne, this was when the reality of the lack of support services for the Sickle Cell community sunk in.

Realizing that they both had the same vision and the same desire for greater awareness and change in the Sickle Cell community, Suzanne and Joyce combined their efforts to revive and enhance the inactive support group, to no avail.

In February 2008, they decided to form their own organization with other like minded parents. They reached out to the Hematology doctors, nurses, and social workers, and families in the Sickle Cell community to formulate strategies for solutions to the problems and lack of support in this area.

In March 2008, they held a meeting with other interested members of the Sickle Cell community, sharing their vision for the organization. In April, they elected board members. At their first board meeting in May, the board developed the mission, goals and vision statements, and a name:

- **F**amily - About our families, for our families affected by this disease.
- **A**dvocacy - To promote and aid in advancement of research and trail studies for a cure.
- **C**oalition - The bringing together of national and local community organizations, medical institutions and

professionals, and our influential African American community leaders and businesses to work toward creating a greater awareness, and changing the stigmas that surround the Sickle Cell community.

- **Empowerment** - By arming the Sickle Cell Community with the education, information, knowledge and its implementation.

www.facefoundationinc,org

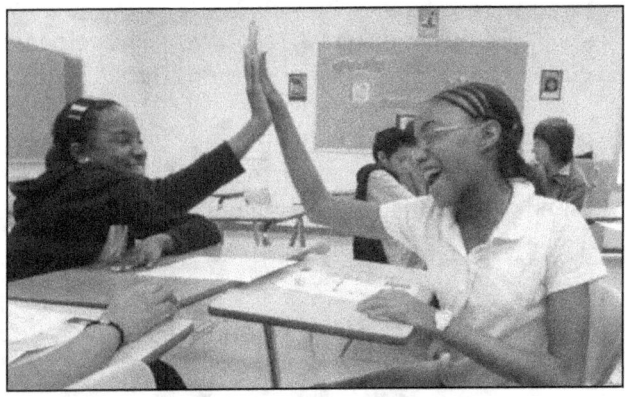

Aaron in celebration of life.

In June 2009 as I searched the internet, a story on the front page caught my attention. There was a picture of a child in a hospital bed surrounded by stuffed animals. In reading the story I would discover the moving story of Jasmina.

Jasmina was an energetic kindergartener in New York. Her mother Theodora Anemia took her to the hospital after a night of severe itching on her foot. On that day, January 20th, Theodora would get the surprise of her life. After several tests including a bone marrow biopsy and finally a spinal tap, her daughter, Jasmina, was diagnosed with Aggressive NK Leukemia. This is a very rare type of leukemia and has been only seen in about thirty cases. Leukemia, cancer of the blood is often referred to as a liquid tumor that just runs through the blood.

The following months for Jasmina and Theodora would be a rollercoaster ride, in and out of the hospital with hopes raised and dashed with consistent uncertainty.

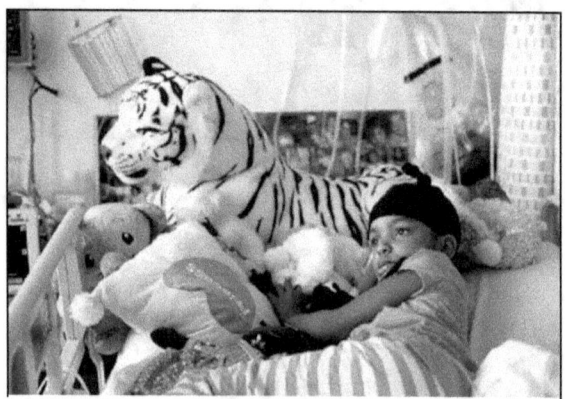

**Jasmine Anema**

As I followed the story it began to take on a powerful life that would ultimately have a tremendous impact on creating awareness for the need to have more donors on the registry.

It would attract local, national and international media as this kindergartener and her mother struggled to find a matching donor to save her life.

Perhaps her story is best told by Theodora and her friend Karen on posts featured on the web site www.carringbridge.org

**Here is Jasmina's Story**

Saturday, January 24, 2009

Isabelle, Wim and Karen spent the day with Jasmina. She was sooooo happy to see her BFF. They played together like usual. Jasmina played tricks on her nurse. She pretended to be asleep when the nurse came in so she would leave her alone. Later, she ran down the hall so Karen had to run after her with the IV stand to keep her tubes from disconnecting. Jasmina wouldn't slow down no matter how loud Karen yelled. It was a very good day.

Monday, January 26, 2009

Sunday was a good day for Jasmina. She is energetic, fiesty and in great spirits. Her response to the chemo protocol is what the doctor was hoping for at this point. He commented that he was relieved that she is feeling so well

Friday, January 30, 2009 9:42 AM, CST

Apparently Jasmina's cancer is so strong that it proved resilient to the first round of chemo. Now she is on an even stronger chemo that is very toxic. Good thing is, as of this morning her white blood cell count went down to 18 from 25. It needs to be at 10, so a little way to go but this last new chemo seems to make some headway. Because of her reduced immunity we are holding off on all unnecessary visitors. She may not eat food brought in from the outside either, so please don't send anything for Jasmina.

Sunday, February 1, 2009

Last night was a rough night. Jasmina's temperature shot up to 104.8. After 2 hours of intense medications, antibiotics, antifungals, horse strength Tylenol etc., her temperature went down. The new chemo protocol, while proving hard on Jasmina's system, has done its job! Her white count went from 25 to 18 to 4.5 to 0.7 in less than 3 days!!! Now her body is at its most vulnerable so PLEASE NO VISITORS WHO ARE AT ALL NOT FEELING WELL OR HAVE BEEN AROUND SOMEONE WHO IS SICK! It is best to wait to visit when Jasmina's immunity is back up..

Thursday, February 5, 2009

Jasmina is doing very well. Her doctor is very happy with her progress. At 7 AM she will have a spinal tap to make sure the Leukemia has not entered her spinal fluid. She will receive another dose of chemo to keep the fluid Leukemia free. The doctor will take a bone marrow sample to see if there is any trace of the Leukemia in Jasmina's marrow. She has started receiving regular transfusions to build up her white cells and platelets

Friday, February 6, 2009

Jasmina is in high spirits today. She got a princess dress in the mail and she looks gorgeous. The results of her spinal tap and bone marrow biopsy are in. The doctor was hoping the leukemia would be gone from her marrow, but it is not. She will definitely need the second round of chemo. Her spinal fluid is still leukemia free so that is really good.

Just so everyone is prepared, Jasmina's hair is due to fall out next week. We ordered wigs almost 2 weeks ago, so hopefully they will arrive on time. If anyone with children plans on visiting, be sure to find out the status of Jasmina's hair beforehand and prepare your children so they don't stare or ask what is wrong with Jasmina's hair in front of her. When she was told her hair would fall out the first thing she said was that the kids at school would make fun of her so please be sensitive to this.

Monday, February 16, 2009 12:11 PM, EST

GREAT NEWS! Jasmina has not had a fever now for 2 days!!! The doctor still does not know the cause of the infection but it looks as if she is through the worst of it! As a matter of fact, her doctor actually said he has never seen a patient who has done this well after being given the aggressive chemotherapy that Jamina has received! Her white blood counts are still very low, making her susceptible to infection, but it looks as if those counts are slowly rising as well! Her mood and energy is terrific!

Jasmina still requires daily blood and platelet transfusions.

Sunday, February 22, 2009

Jasmina is still as energetic and spunky as ever...She is still extremely neutropenic but has no infection anymore. She had another bone marrow biopsy that revealed leukemia cells still in her marrow. Because the leukemia is so aggressive, she will be starting the second round of chemotherapy on Monday. Unfortunately she will not be going home anytime soon and will celebrate her 6th birthday in the hospital.

Jasmina had a visit this week from the hair fairy! She left Jasmina $1 for each of her braids...totaling $108 dollars! Jasmina no longer has her hair but is enjoying her new wigs. She also seems to be having odd cravings for food and has Thea running out all hours to find things like salami! Friday the hospital had some NFL players visit the children's floor. The players were so tall and big that Jasmina got scared and hid under her bed! She is still feisty and fun and continues her activities in the hospital (school, play, movies, reading, music, and keeping the doctors and nurses on their toes!)

Friday, February 27, 2009

Thursday was a busy, exciting day. Jasmina had a bone marrow biopsy this morning. The results were disappointing. While the leukemia levels in her blood have gone down, the leukemia load in her marrow has increased. This means that while the chemotherapy has helped her clinical well being, it has not reduced her leukemia. She started her new chemo protocol today. They injected chemo into her bones and are giving it to her through her port as well. It is a new medication, so hopefully the leukemia responds to this one and GOES AWAY! I know this sounds discouraging, but for some reason, I have no doubt that everything will be fine in the end. Jasmina is still strong and vivacious and happy which means we have time to get the chemo cocktail right and I believe we will.

Now for the exciting part...... Today, Chris Wilcox of the NY Nicks, came by to see Jasmina. After several minutes of hiding under the bed, Jasmina was coaxed out and convinced to stay in her bed for a photo op by her stuffed dog, Jackie. Jackie told Jasmina that her favorite basketball player is Chris and that even though Chris was coming to take a picture with Jasmina, she hoped that Jasmina would hold her so she could be in the picture too. Jasmina promised Jackie she could be in the photo and she kept her promise. Chris arrived and Jasmina had the best time with him. He brought her a pink build a bear which he named Hope. He brought clothes for it and "glass" slippers with high heels. Chris even dressed the bear for Jasmina. He was so sweet and so cute with her. He tickled her and hugged her and she loved it.

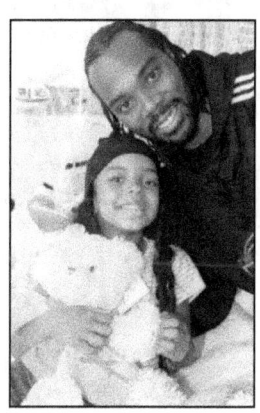

Jasmina and NBA star Chris Wilcox

Monday, February 23, 2009

The protocol will take one month to complete, at which time Dr. Carroll will decide if Jasmina is ready for a transplant already or if they need to do another month of chemo after this one. If there is no match, they will do the 3rd round of chemo while they are waiting for a match. That means we have 1 to 1 1/2 months more to find a match. If none is found in the bone marrow registry or at the donor drive, Jasmina will receive a cord blood stem cell transplant instead of receiving a bone marrow transplant.

Wednesday, March 4, 2009

Today was Jasmina's 6th BIRTHDAY and what a birthday it was! She had a fashion show runway party complete with red carpet runway with foot lights. Kelly Rowland of Destiny's child hung out with Jasmina for a couple of hours and sang Happy Birthday to her.

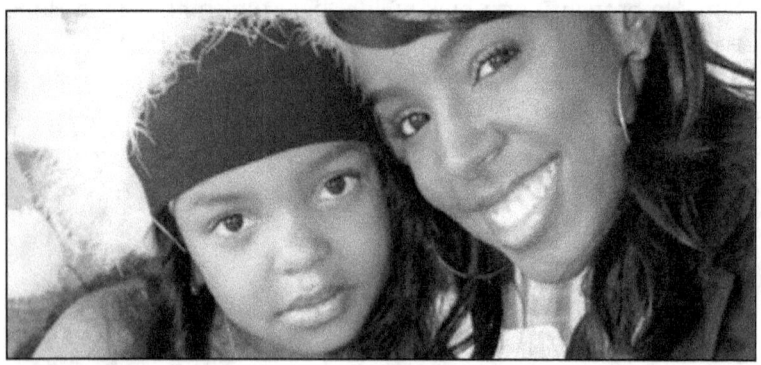

Jasmine and Kelly Rowland

The news crews where stuffed into Jasmina's room trying to get the scoop. Jasmina was quite the center of attention. After everyone left, Jasmina and Isabelle decorated cupcakes to give to Jasmina's favorite doctors and nurses. Despite painful sores in her mouth, she managed to eat several cupcakes.

Thursday, March 5, 2009

GREAT NEWS>>> Jasmina had her bone marrow biopsy today and the leukemia load has gone from 36% down to 22%!!!!!!!!! And the leukemia is taking on characteristics which are more like t-cells instead of aggressive natural killer cells which is also good. Dr. Carroll will continue with this chemo protocol.

Do to the popularity of Jasmina's story, ONEFORJASMINA.com, crashed because we used up all the server space on the Eastern seaboard!! Jasmina is everywhere. We were the lead story on AOL.com for most of the day which contributed to the crash.

Tuesday, March 24, 2009

We had a very unfortunate day today, as we found out the results of Jasmina's weekly bone marrow biopsy. While the last round of chemotherapy brought her leukemia marrow count down to 8%, it has climbed back up and is now at 30%. That is even higher than when she was initially brought into the hospital.

Jasmina was moved to Sloan Kettering last week in hopes of starting the transplant process. She actually spent the weekend at home, running and dancing around her apartment, sleeping in her own bed and taking a bath in her own bathtub! All without an IV!

Today, after discovering these new results she was readmitted to NYU and is again under the care of Dr. Carroll. She is in room 965. She will be starting a new chemotherapy treatment tomorrow, which will hopefully be more effective, so we can get the transplant process moving. Jasmina, amazingly, still remains in good spirits!

Wednesday, April 8, 2009

Tonight Jasmina was on Access Hollywood! Rihanna visited Jasmina in the hospital last week where they spent hours doing makeovers and manicures

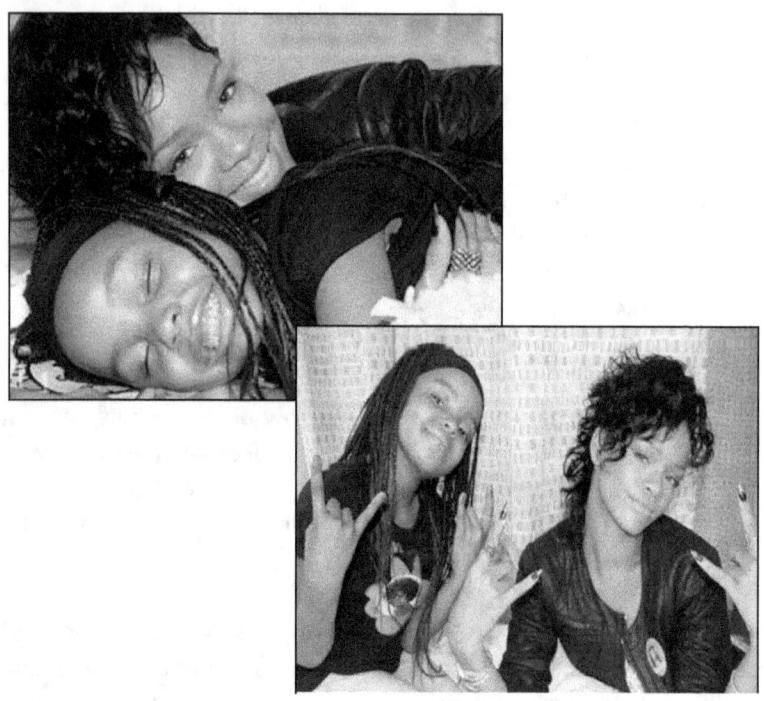

Jasmina and Rihanna

Jasmina's story has reached so many people. Over 12,000 donors have registered into the world wide banks trying to help Jasmina find the perfect marrow match. Thank you to everyone who has helped by becoming a donor or by spreading the word!

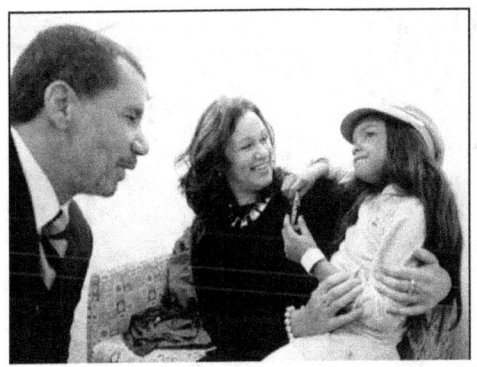

New York Governor, David A. Paterson

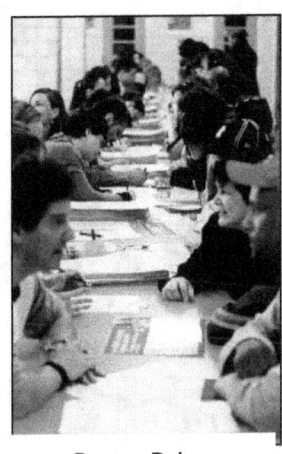

Donor Drive

We are still waiting on the results of the recent drives to find a match for Jasmina

On an AMAZING note, while there were no matches for Jasmina from the PS41 drive, there is a perfect match for a 38 year old patient who is in need of a donor!! Thanks to Jasmina and her supporters, he has a chance to be saved!

Sunday, April 12, 2009

HAPPY EASTER Everyone! Jasmina had a bone marrow biopsy on Thursday and her numbers are GOOD!!!!!!! This means that the leukemia is finally getting weak in response to the most recent chemo she had. Jasmina is out of the hospital for the Easter weekend. She is spending the weekend at Isabelle's house.

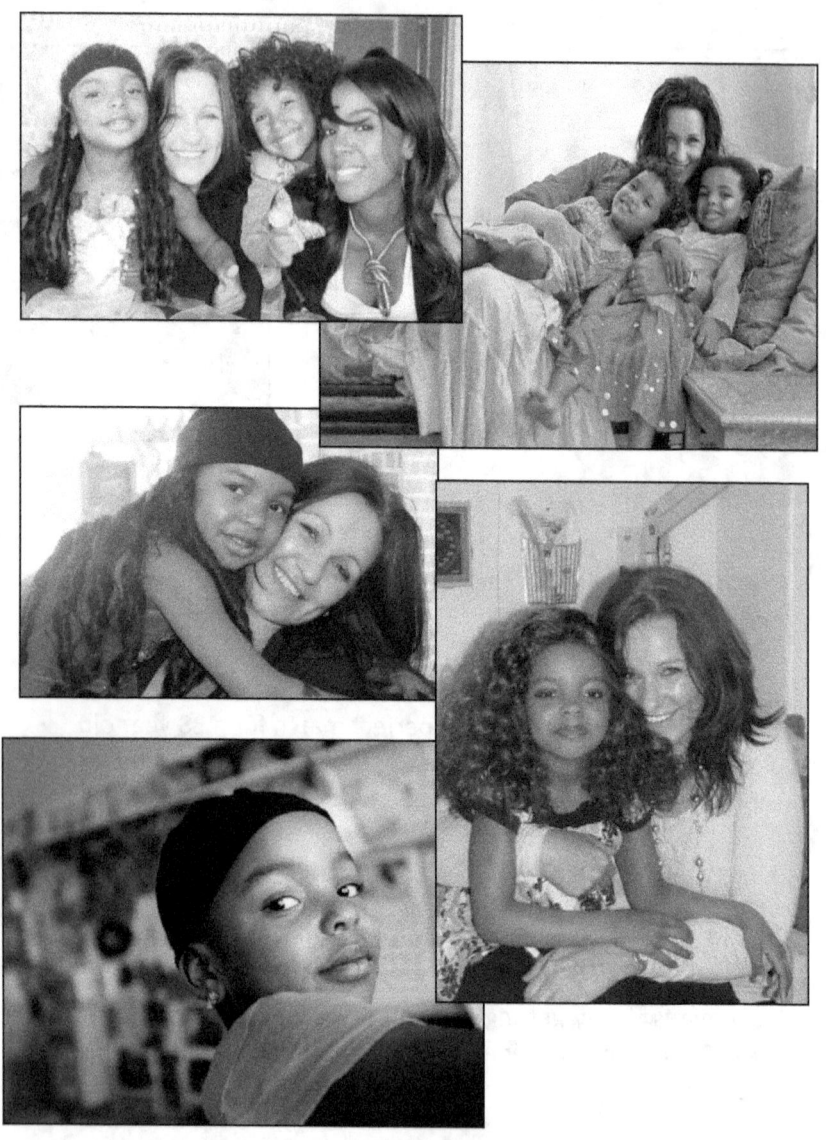

Friday, May 1, 2009

AMAZING, AMAZING, AMAZING NEWS!!! Jasmina's biopsy went well and the leukemia in her bone marrow is 0%!!!!!!!!!!!!!!!!!!!

This means that she is eligible for a transplant as soon as her blood levels recover. The doctors will do another biopsy next week to check that the leukemia level is staying low.

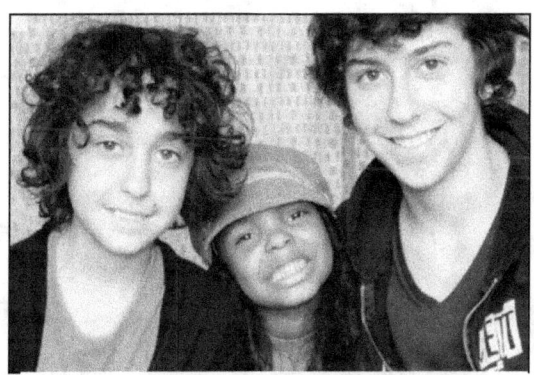

Jasmina and the Naked Brothers

On Wednesday, the Naked Brothers paid Jasmina a visit. They were totally delightful and Jasmina and Isabelle played with them for over an hour. They autographed pictures for the girls and then signed a huge stack of photos to give to all the other kids on the floor.

Today Jasmina received a gift of a special photo shoot where she was transformed into the celebrity of her choice. No, not Rihanna. Not Gwen Stefani. Yes, Beyonce!! What a diva she was and she even got to keep the wig.

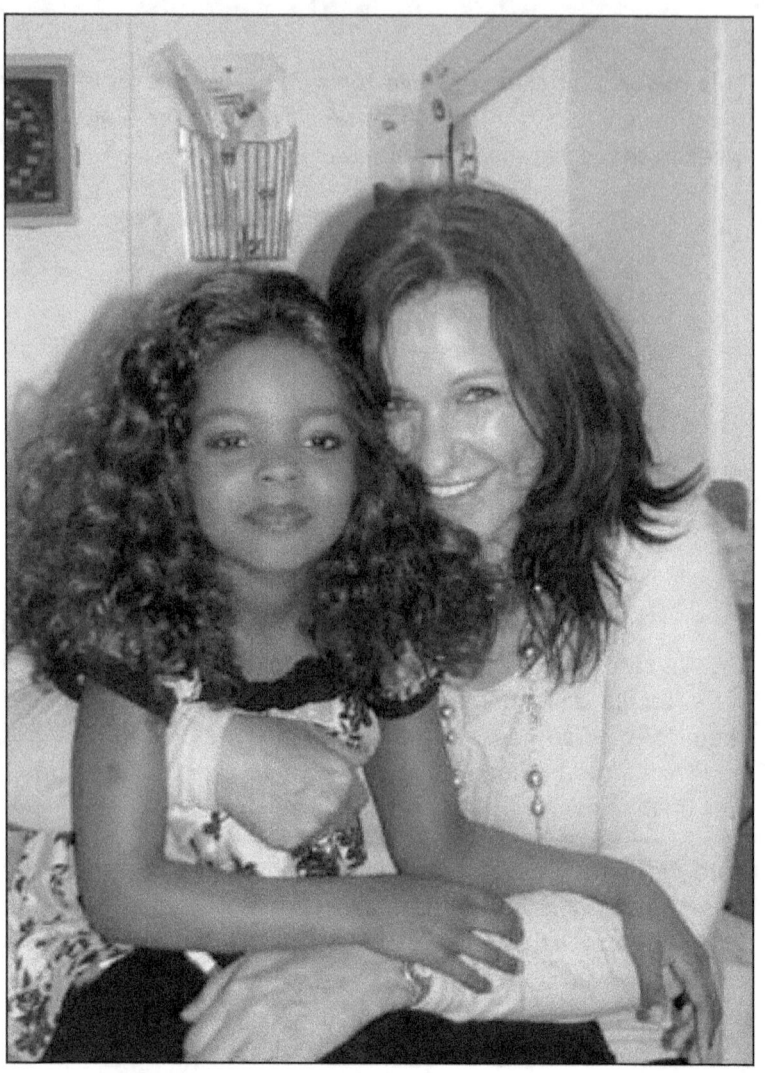

Wednesday, May 6, 2009

Great news....two 9 out of 10 matches have been found for Jasmina! As long as her counts remain good she will move to transplant mid-May.

If Jasmina's platelet counts are high enough tomorrow (currently they are not) she will have a bone marrow biopsy to determine if the leukemia cells are still low enough for transplant. She is receiving platelets today in hopes of raising her count.

Also, to clarify what this "zero" count means, the leukemia is not detected in her marrow but still may be present in her body. Due to its aggressive nature it may also have grown back over the last week...SO, if the leukemia count is low enough she will then go to Sloan to start transplant next week.

The process of transplant is actually harder than anything Jasmina has faced so far. The levels of radiation and chemotherapy she will be receiving are extremely strong and very toxic. Because Jasmina has been so "clinically healthy" through this process, the doctors really feel that she get through the transplant process. We are very fortunate to have made it through so many rounds of chemotherapy and still have a healthy little girl! So, the radiation and chemotherapy will be about a three week process, followed by transplant and then another month or so of recovery.

Before transplant, the two donors still need to pass medical clearance. Because the match is not 100%, there is a chance of Jasmina's body rejecting the bone marrow. This is called Graft-vs-Host disease. The doctor's have never seen anyone tolerate chemotherapy like Jasmina and have high hopes that this will not happen. But, it is always a possibility.

Over the past few months Thea's friend and now detective, Mariana, has done some pretty serious discovery work! She was able to locate and arrange a meeting for Thea to meet Jasmina's birth mother and extended family. They flew down to Virginia this past weekend and met 30 family members. Thea swabbed the entire family as possible donors for Jasmina. She most likely will not find a full match there but they want to cover all bases for Jasmina. There are some hospitals that are doing experimental partial transplants, so she wanted to test everyone "just in case"!

Friday, May 8, 2009

Today we have the results from Jasmina's bone marrow biopsy. Unfortunately, the leukemia is proving to be extremely aggressive and it grows back very quickly. Jasmina currently has about 20% of the bone marrow in her body that a healthy person has. Of that 20%, 10% of her bone marrow has leukemia. In one week's time it has come back, and needs to be treated immediately. The doctor's have consulted and have agreed to go ahead with the transplant, even though her count is higher than it should be.

**Next steps:**

Jasmina moves to Sloan Kettering next Monday or Tuesday. She then begins preparation for radiation and chemotherapy. Once she starts chemo and radiation, she will be in isolation and there will be very strict rules for her care, for visitation, food, etc. The treatment is VERY AGGRESSIVE and will take about 2 and a half weeks. She will then have a day's rest and then the transplant happens. Once she gets the bone marrow transplant, the doctors expect a 2 to 3 week recovery. She will be watched closely to make sure her body does not reject the new marrow. So, if all goes as planned she could potentially return home sometime in June.

Again, as has been all along, Jasmina is clinically very healthy. Her energy is great! She eats well (even if she sometimes has cupcakes for breakfast)! She sings, dances, reads, draws, goes to school, plays, teases, laughs endlessly, and sometimes even does gymnastics around the room...

So, all in all, she is mentally and physically in a very good place to start the transplant process. Again, the doctors believe that this will help her to come through the difficult procedures she now faces.

Let me start off by saying I am truly amazed every day by Jasmina. Every step along the way of this difficult journey has been met with energy, laughter, goofiness and determination. From her little chants of "I can do it, I can do it" when having to take medicine or receive shots, to her joking with the entire nursing staff to her near gymnastics around the hospital room, she never ceases to amaze me and those around her! She is so happy and so loving, even through all that has happened...she is a little miracle!

Tuesday, May 12, 2009

We had some very disappointing news yesterday. Jasmina has developed some lesions on her head over the past few days that the doctors have identified as Shingles. Very simply put, Shingles is a painful rash that is caused by the same virus that causes chicken pox. Once a person has had chickenpox, the virus can live, but remain inactive, in certain nerve roots within the body. If it becomes active again, usually later in life, it can cause Shingles. Jasmina did not catch Shingles from anyone. Shingles tends to happen if a person's immune system has been compromised, as we know hers has been.

Shingles typically stay in one nerve area, and on Jasmina, they are on her head. She only has a few, so as of now she is not really uncomfortable. Hopefully she won't suffer from any pain or itching. What is difficult, though, is that she is confined to her bed, which is encased in a large plastic tent. Air is being circulated though the tent to help dry up the lesions. She is contagious to anyone who has not had the chicken pox or who has not had an immunization.

Unfortunately, because of the Shingles, she will not be able to start the transplant process at Sloan. She will most likely be at NYU now for another 2 weeks where she will be treated for the Shingles.

She will also need treatment for the leukemia as well, as it is extremely fast growing. Even though it is not ideal while she has Shingles, she MUST receive chemotherapy as her leukemia count has increased 50% in one week. The doctors will wait two days to see if her condition of Shingles worsens and then begin chemo.

Thankfully Jasmina is still feeling well. She was busy this weekend with a few visits from friends. She has also been having virtual visits via computer. She is quite a little actress as she poses and goofs around in front of the camera. We are hoping that this setback does not affect her too drastically. As you can imagine, it could prove to be very difficult for her to be so confined.

The emotional roller coaster of this entire experience has taken its toll on Thea. All of your support and love is needed now more than ever. Stay tuned, we will keep you updated as soon as we have more details.

Saturday, May 16, 2009

Jasmina has approached this battle as she would her everyday life...with optimism, joy, cheerfulness and without fear. When I am faced with the challenges of my day to day life I think of Jasmina and the attitude she brings to this problem. She lives right here, right now, grounded in the present moment, not worrying about all of what could or might happen. Even through pain and through physical limitations she is the same spark plug she was before, laughing and smiling and being truly delightful!

Tuesday, June 2, 2009

**Today is a very big day for Jasmina!** She has her first 2 doses of radiation-the process has officially begun. She had a bone marrow biopsy and her lines were changed today as well. We get the results from everything later today and tomorrow. She has the radiation treatments 3 times a day for 40 minutes each-standing up in a small tube-like room-not moving...it's going to be really tough. Radiation is the most difficult thing she has gone through so far, so we will keep you informed as to how she does with it. Side effects vary from person to person-it can affect every organ in her body, and we won't know if the damage is permanent. It could stunt her growth as well. But, it will also get rid of the NASTY leukemia and prepare her for her transplant- so we are all keeping a very positive outlook, and trying to follow her optimistic approach to life!!! She is looking forward to going home, to the summer, to catching butterflies and smelling the fresh air...and of course to getting her new kitty cat, Lucky!

The rest of the transplant process is simplified as follows: Radiation now through Saturday, 3 times a day.

Then she will have 4 days of chemotherapy.

On 6/10 the donor marrow will be harvested

6/11-TRANSPLANT DAY!!!!!!!!!!!!!!!!!!!!

On 6/12, 6/14, 6/17, 6/22 she will receive more chemotherapy. Then if all goes well, and she does not get graph versus host disease, she should be able to go home the end of the month or beginning July.

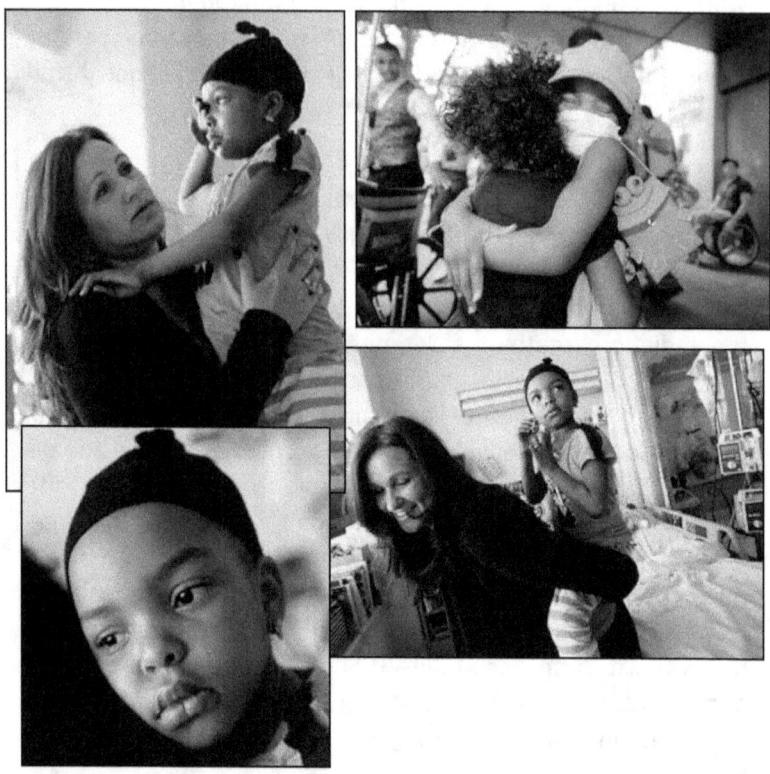

All this week Jasmina has be getting her preliminary transplant tests. It was determined yesterday that her shingles are still active. Because this means Jasmina is contagious, she has been moved to isolation on the 5th floor at Sloan. Her full body radiation was scheduled to begin, Tuesday May 27th. Now, due to the active shingles, this may be delayed. At this point it is a waiting game. She could be free of the virus by Tuesday and begin on schedule, or it could take longer until she is virus free.

When she does begin radiation, it will be administered 3 times a day for 4 days. The radiation happens in a machine like a MRI machine, except that Jasmina is standing up for 40 minutes at a time. This is very difficult so we are hoping that she can manage this. Immediately following the days of radiation, she will receive chemo for several days.

After this, the room will be prepared for "after transplant". The walls, bed, chairs etc. will be sterilized and all belongings have to leave the room and need to be thoroughly sanitized before coming back in. NO stuffed animals allowed.

If she begins the full body radiation on schedule (starting Tuesday) she will receive her transplant, Thursday 6/4. After that she will get more chemo but only every other day. Then approximately 30 days from transplant day, depending on complications, she should be ready to go home where she will need to be isolated for 6 months and will receive home schooling. During these six months, she will receive outpatient care 3 times a week.

After the 6 month period ends, Jasmina will need to get all her childhood vaccinations again because the immunity she received from her previous vaccines will have been destroyed by the transplant radiation.

Please pray for a quick recovery from the shingles so Jasmina can get on with the transplant and remain on a speedy schedule to recovery. Like Jasmina says after a prayer; "GOD, thank you for your cooperation".

Wednesday, June 10, 2009

**The big day is finally here!!!!** Jasmina will receive her long awaited bone marrow transplant this Thursday!!!!! HURRAY!!!!! The bone marrow was harvested on Tuesday, is being sent over to Sloan on Wednesday and transplanted on Thursday to our wonderful Jasmina!!! She and her mom are ecstatic!

The actual transplant is much easier for Jasmina than the rest of the process has been. She will basically hang out in her bed on Thursday afternoon where the marrow will go directly into her lines. It takes only a few hours!

Three weeks from transplant she will have another bone marrow biopsy to see if there is any possible leukemia left. During this time the healthy "new" bone marrow will be generating new cells for Jasmina. We can only hope that the radiation and now 11 rounds of chemotherapy have killed off all the leukemia cells, making way for this fresh bone marrow to do its magic. We will know in approximately 1 month from transplant how her body reacts to the new marrow and whether or not she accepts or rejects it.

Right now Jasmina is hooked up to some pretty serious machines. She gets antibiotics daily as well as constant fluids, nutrition and pain medication. On the days following the radiation, Jasmina received two chemotherapy treatments.

The first was really difficult in that it required Jasmina to be scrubbed down until her skin was red every six hours-even in the middle of the night. The chemo was excreted through her skin and needed to be scrubbed away. Jasmina described the whole thing as "ouchy".

The second chemo was very dangerous for her liver, so she was given tons of extra fluids to flush it out of her body and liver. As you can imagine she is up and down to the bathroom constantly even all through the night. Unfortunately she occasionally has had accidents making night time quite a challenge.

We are not sure whether it is the chemo or the radiation, or both, but Jasmina has no appetite right now. She is being given nutrition through the IV but she has not eaten any food for a full week now. Actually, I take that back, she ate 1 piece of popcorn last night. And then she held the cup of popcorn tightly clutched to her side while she napped for several hours. She has expressed interest in bologna, sausage and pop tarts, but when she actually gets them she has no desire to eat. We hope her appetite returns soon.

Jasmina still has some pain from the shingles, but mostly now it's more of an irritating itching on her head. Her eye is still almost swollen shut. Her skin color has changed slightly, becoming darker and gray. Her energy level has decreased substantially and she sleeps a lot more than she used to, sometimes sleeping in 'til almost noon!

When she's not asleep, Jasmina can be found doing school work. The teachers cannot believe she is only in kindergarten. She is reading at the fifth grade level and is writing beautifully. She has even learned to write her name in cursive. She also has become extremely fond of scrabble and plays it quite frequently.

Jasmina also plays Wii when she has the energy. During transplant it is important for patients to stay active and get exercise. She gets hers by playing tennis, bowling and boxing. She says boxing is her favorite!!! Of course she loves all the princess games too!

Thursday, June 11, 2009

**Today was THE DAY!!!!!** Jasmina finally received her bone marrow transplant today. It started at 11:15 this morning and lasted until 1:45 this afternoon. It was a fairly simple process and went very well. It's incredible to realize that Jasmina's flesh and blood will soon be from a complete stranger. She can now celebrate 2 birthdays, her original one and one that marks the day that her body developed from yet another human being... AMAZING!

Jasmina's marrow donor will remain anonymous for the first year. We are extremely grateful that this wonderful person has helped our "little princess" to have a healthy, happy life! THANK YOU!!!!!

Jasmina feels fine, and at the moment she is knitting a scarf for her stuffed dog "Jackie". She just learned how to knit yesterday and is already making something! She's taking orders for sweaters next!

Today has been a media frenzy! After Jasmina's transplant story appeared in the newspaper yesterday, the news channels have been calling like crazy. No one was allowed in the room so Thea did interviews outside, in front of the hospital. Channel 1, 2, 4 and 5 interviewed Thea. Channel 7 and 11 contacted the PR department of the hospital but the hospital declined. Keep your eyes open for the wonderful story!

As you can imagine, we are **ecstatic** to say the least. "On top of the world" is a little closer to how happy we are that this day has come. We want to thank everyone who has been there along the way, to get us to this point. Without the support from wonderful friends and family, this journey would have been even harder than it has been. Thank you to all of the supporters who have come forth and shared time, love and resources. The outpour of support that we have witnessed over the past months is truly incredible! Thank you to all of the wonderful staff at NYU who helped Jasmina in so many ways. Thank you to the excellent doctors who have been a vital part of her care. And thank you to everyone at Sloan for continuing with the treatments and the transplant! We owe you **ALL** more thanks than is possible to express in words!

Jasmina is officially engrafted as of last Sunday but it take 100 days from transplant (June 11) before she will be free of possible G vs. HD (graft versus host disease). She'll need to take medication to prevent G vs. HD for up to one year. They are weaning her slowly off some of the antibiotics and changing some to oral doses in anticipation of her going home. The doctors are extremely pleased with her progress. Her organs, such as her liver, show no damage from the radiation. She has a few mouth sores but nothing terrible. Yesterday she drank two sips of water... the first in a month. She still has no appetite and no sense of taste, so she has not eaten in over a month.

Friday, June 26, 2009

This week has been one of healing and resting for Jasmina. She is now 2 weeks out of transplant and is slowly getting better. She no longer has a stomach infection and her morphine doses have been lowered since she does not suffer from as much pain. Jasmina, however, is still not eating or drinking. The fancy combinations of chemo and radiation have squashed her appetite and taste buds. She is being fed intravenously though so she is not losing any weight. She is actually gaining weight since this "nutrition" has so many calories.

Jasmina's eye is still closed but we have been assured that there is no damage to the eye. It is just still very sensitive from the shingles. In another week or so she should be able to open it comfortably. She has some blotchy patches on her skin, and her skin is several shades darker than normal. This is from the radiation and the chemo that was excreted through her skin. It should also minimize over the next several months.

Jasmina is receiving a new medication to raise her white blood counts which are currently at zero. She also receives platelets and blood transfusions every other day. She received her last dose of chemo for awhile just 2 days ago. Her body is making new healthy cells every day. Next week is her bone marrow biopsy to determine if there is any leukemia in her marrow. And then a week after that we should know if her body has accepted the transplant.

In the meantime she is just being a kid. She is cheerful and goofy as always. She spends her day sleeping and cuddling her mama. Sometimes she sleeps so much in the day that she stays up 'til all hours of the night. Needless to say, Thea's a bit tired!! She tells Thea over and over "Mama, I am sooo happy that you are my mama!! I love you soooo much".

She had her last day of school on Wednesday and is officially on summer vacation. She ended the year reading several years ahead of where most kids her age are... and was also doing double digit math calculations! AMAZING! She still has her amazing sense of humor and is constantly saying the funniest things...when she needs to be awakened to be weighed or for a doctor's visit she says "don't wake me up, I'm trying to dream!"

Friday, July 24, 2009

It's time to celebrate! Today, after 6 long months in the hospital, Jasmina finally went home! She was greeted outside the hospital by Isabelle and her mom, and several news teams!

The results of the bone marrow biopsy were also very good! A nurse will come to the house with an IV pole and to teach Thea how to care for Jasmina medically. Thea is so excited to play in her new role as Nurse Thea! Jasmina will receive 12 hours of fluids at night to keep her hydrated. She had several medications as well. But, she is home, in her happy place! And that is more than enough reason for everyone to celebrate today!!!!

Monday, August 3, 2009

Written by Thea...

It is about time I write an update myself... so here is the latest.
It has not been easy this past weekend-a lot of throwing up, diarrhea and ridiculously high blood pressure. I was afraid that this was a sign of transplant rejection but thank goodness it is not
I have been going thru a bit of an emotional time. This Dutch magazine needed some photos of her so I came across all these images from a year ago where she exhibits the epitome of health, happiness and energy. Comparing to today's state, it was just so hard to realize that the once so lively, beautiful and healthy child is now only awake a few hours a day, not eating, her left eye mostly closed, her head and partial face covered with markings from the shingles, her arms tainted from all the needles and her long braids gone.

Anyway, I am glad the fever is gone and they found the cause. She still has a very high blood pressure and receives medication for this and needs to stay on antibiotics for a week. So maybe next week we can finally go home, let's keep our fingers crossed.
I want to thank all the well wishers for their continuously sweet and encouraging messages on this site.
Thank you so much,
Jasmina and Thea

Saturday, July 25, 2009

Yesterday was one of the happiest days for Thea and Jasmina and everyone who loves them! Isabelle and Jasmina played, danced, ate candy, went on a pretend trip and ran naked through the house giggling and squealing while we enjoyed their laughter! We had the best time watching the girls be together after such a long time. A visiting nurse taught Thea how to hook Jasmina up to her medications via I.V. lines which she did all by herself last night for the first time.

Jasmina got a bit of a fever last night around 11:00PM. We monitored her for about an hour before deciding that is was not the excitement making her hot. We took her back to the hospital as a standard precaution. She will now have to be monitored full-time in the hospital for 3-5 days. This is typical for patients with severely compromised immune systems. This will probably not be the last time she will have to return to the hospital over the next several months. It's just a bummer that it happened at the peak of her happy homecoming. Thea is understandably BUMMED OUT and Jasmina was pretty angry when she realized she would not be treated and released last night. By 6:00AM she was over it and was asking for paper and pens so she could make drawings. She is truly amazing.

Wednesday, August 12, 2009

Last Friday Jasmina had another MRI of her head to make sure there is no nerve damage since her eye still does not fully open. The result was good. The MRI looked perfect. The doctors took her off the antibiotics last Friday and kept her in the hospital for the weekend to make sure her fever did not come back like twice before. It did not, HOORAY!!! So the plan was to go home either Sunday or Monday. In preparation for her return home, the doctors changed a lot of her medications to pill form instead of liquid. She takes the pills mixed with pudding, but since she hasn't eaten very much for the last 3 months, she immediately throws up and we have to repeat the medication. Plus it's very difficult to give a sleeping child an oral medication.

Then her level of fascarnet was too high so the doctors lowered her dose and decided to monitor her for a few days which postponed our return home to Wednesday. But now Jasmina is literally sleeping all day long. She is only awake for 2 or 3 hours a day and when she is awake, she has absolutely no energy. Yesterday she played her Nintendo game, which she usually plays for hours, but after 15 minutes she fell asleep again. Since she is still not eating, except for some of my friends special chicken soup sporadically, the doctors told me this morning that there is no way we can go home. She is thankfully not in pain, just lethargic and a far cry from 2 weeks ago when we went home for a few hours. The doctors think this might be because of

lack of nutrition or depression. They have her back on TPN, the IV nutrition. I am not convinced it is lack of nutrition or depression as a doctor suggested. She tells me that she feels fine, just sleepy but on the other hand, I need to constantly lay next to her and hold and caress her because she is just not herself.

Tomorrow they will do another bone marrow biopsy and a spinal fluid tap to see if an infection is lingering in her system even though she does not have a fever.

GOOD NEWS FLASH. . . Today Jasmina's doctor asked Thea if there was anything she thought might cheer Jasmina up. Thea responded that the only thing she could think of was Isabelle, so the doctor approved a special BFF visit. Isabelle brought Jasmina a hula skirt, coconut bra, shell necklace and fake flower lei as a present from Hawaii. She arrived just in time for Jasmina's Dance Therapy session. The girls hula danced in bed and Karen and the therapist danced around the room while Thea laughed on. Jasmina ate a box of Cheerios and two small servings of chicken soup while Isabelle was there. When the doctor came in and saw how happy Jasmina was she decided that there is no "underlying problem" and cancelled the exploratory marrow fluid tap which was scheduled for the morning. After a brief two hour visit from Isabelle, a very happy Jasmina floated off to sleep. Thea is very happy that Little Ms. Prozac stopped by. It was just the medicine Jasmina needed.

Friday, August 21, 2009.

Okay let's start with the good news. The results of Monday's test are fantastic. 0% leukemia and all other cells look like normal growing cells. Her hair is slowly starting to grow back, which demonstrates her recovery...it's an eighth of an inch long!

In the future, she will get 5 more spinal chemo doses as a preventative measure to lower the risk of relapse. She received a Intravenous immunoglobulin transfusion to boost her immune cells. She is still in a lot of pain and the soreness from her feeding tube ( G-tube) in her belly prevents her from talking and moving. She has now been for two straight days in the same position since everything hurts.

Needless to say, we are not going home yet.

Thursday, August 27, 2009

From Thea...

Good news, according to the doctor's, the transplant is so far successful!!!!! Her pain is less after they took the stitches out from her G-tube. She had four long wires poking in her body, so no wonder every little move was hurting. So Now I can finally cuddle her again after abstaining for a week. We made her get up and walk on Monday. Her heels were hurting because she did not walk for such a long period so she could only walk very slowly on her tippy toes. The next day she did 6 rounds in the hallway. Yesterday about 10 without any issues and even said "faster mama, FASTER!!"

Getting this nutrition is definitely getting her energy back which is great. It is fantastic to hear her talk and laugh again and I see slowly the sparkle in her eyes returning.   Her left eye is now 3/4 open and looking a lot better.

Her hair is growing really fast now, soft and sticking straight up kind of what a baby elephant feels and looks like.  It is so surreal to hear people say, "Oh, WOW, your hair is sooo long!!!" while it is only 3/16". Next week probably 1/4". (I am thinking extensions already, HA!) But this rapid hair growth is a side effect from the Tacrolimus. This is the medication to prevent Graft versus Host disease, or transplant rejection if you will.

I miss her voice, her spirit, her laugh etc.

Saturday, September 5, 2009

From Thea

Okay, the most fantastic thing has happened. We are HOME!!!. We came home Thursday late afternoon with a car full of hospital equipment. The last week was tough because she had the most terrible stomach cramps a few times at night together with the painful G-tube. She needed an ultra sound of her kidneys but nothing seemed out of the ordinary, her liver function went back to normal and her feeding went up to 40 ML an hour so we were able to finally be discharged. I need to increase this slowly up to 100ML and we are already up to 50ML without throwing up. We are home with a pole where her feeding and its machine are attached to and I have become an expert nurse, hooking her up, flushing her lines, administering medications every six hours. etc. I even know how to replace her tube in case it is accidently pulled out of her tummy. And of course Jasmina is an excellent nurse assistant pushing her own syringes. I wanted to make sure that this time we were to stay home before updating this site. It has been over 48 hours and she is doing AMAZING!!!! The moment we came home, she miraculously does not have pain anymore (finally I can give her hugs!!!) and the nightly cramps are in the past.!!!. Now she is laughing, playing dress-up, dancing and doing Wii sport. It is so incredible good to see her dancing again. So alive and full of energy!!! YES, she is BACK !!!!! Her left eyelid is still a bit swollen, her face scarred on the left from the shingles (this will be gone before she is a teenager) but otherwise looking almost as if nothing happened. Her hair is now over a 1/4" long and with dress up earrings and her beautifully shaped head, she looks surprisingly sophisticated!! We even went outside for walks. As long as she does not touch anything, keep her mouth and nose covered, we avoid crowds and wash our hands diligently upon return, this is fine. She is not comfortable yet to go in the street with her cropped coif so she wears one of her wigs. Picture her, with movie star sunglasses, a mask, a crazy outfit and her feeding lines sticking out from her clothes to a bag I carry, it is quite a sight. She talks every day about the cat she is going to receive when the doctors give the green light and is full with excitement talking about this and loves the hot pink bed I made for our hopefully soon to be feline room- mate.

Wednesday, September 16, 2009

I took Jasmina to the country this past weekend because the booklet tells me that fresh air is really important. Today, Tuesday my neighbor Jill, asked Jasmina how she liked it upstate after not having been there for 8 months. Her reply; " It is like a dream from the heart" !! Oh my..... My neighbor started crying and it is indeed hard to imagine that this kid is that deep but then again, since she came into my life there are sooooo many things she has expressed that go beyond my wildest imagination. All is well so far. Tomorrow, Wednesday we go for another bone marrow biopsy and let's all keep our fingers crossed that the results be as hope for.

Her first week home has been good. No fevers. Everyday there is some throwing up but nothing alarming. Still not eating but I am managing the feeding tube pretty well. It is almost like sleeping in the Hospital. The machine starts beeping, it is medicine time, her feeding tube hurts, the throwing up and every night she has these intense nightmares where you just cannot wake her up to come out of it. After the procedures on Wednesday we will go upstate again, only coming to the city for Hospital appointments, so she can smell flowers and catch butterflies ( with a mask and gloves) before I will go back to the office on the 24th which I am truly looking forward to.

Saturday, September 19, 2009

Okay, so Wednesday she was supposed to get her bone marrow biopsy and I know of course that you cannot eat the night before prior to anesthesia and I did not give her anything. So there we were 6.30 AM in the hospital when I realized I still had her attached to her feeding tube not realizing that that is food also. In my simple mind food only goes thru the mouth..AAAGGHH !!!

Needless to say, we had to postpone the procedure and received other treatments instead.

Wednesday, September 23, 2009

Again today, Jasmina's numbers were not good. The complete report on her bone marrow came back and the news is devastating. 72% of the marrow cells in the sample they took last week are leukemia cells and not healthy donor cells. Because she is less than six months post transplant, aggressive chemo and a second transplant are not options at this time. It seems that the most likely option for Jasmina is a mild steroid/chemo combo which may be able to keep the leukemia under control until we are closer to being able to do another bone marrow transplant about three months from now. The doctors are discouraged because she came out of remission so early after the transplant and her numbers are increasing so rapidly. Both of these things are indicators that the leukemia is still acting very aggressively and will be difficult to overcome. The only thing good I can say is that Isabelle and Jasmina played Wii baseball today and were giggling and swinging their bats like it was the most fun they've ever had. Tonight they are having a sleep over just like the good old days. It's really nice to see.

Tuesday, September 29, 2009

From Thea. Okay, I suppose it is time I write something myself. Post transplant everything was going great and I kept fantasizing about going back to our normal life very soon. It started with the feeding tube- Nothing but agony and pain. Besides that, it only caused throwing up and diarrhea. She became lethargic, no energy and always tired. I became so frustrated that I took her of the feeds, a chemically induced formula. I boiled some organic broccoli, mixed it with my friend's Elaine's homemade chicken stock, liquefied it in the blender, funneled it into a fat syringe and transferred it straight into her tummy through the feeding tube. It stayed in. Later I did the same with spinach, carrots and more organic chicken. She was no longer attached to a pole, hooking her up to the machine and no more calculating the ML's per hour, etc. Free to walk around, play and so on. I was honest with the doctors about it they told me to keep doing what I was doing. We were last Wednesday in the hospital. her counts had gone down so she received a blood transfusion and a medication to boost her counts. Friday the bone marrow biopsy and more blood-work- The counts were lower than Wednesday. Saturday we went back and the counts were again lower then Friday and she needed platelets. Even though we were supposed to be outpatient, we spent almost every day in the hospital. Transfusions, meds, ultrasounds and an x-ray of her feeding tube because I insisted that something would be terribly wrong otherwise she could not be in that much pain. No one can go near it, she walks crooked and keeps a cupped hand over it to protect it. Even when I have to lift her up, I can only do so if she holds my neck and I put my arm behind her knees. All this uncertainty was wearing on me.

So last Monday, her counts were again lower and I was told her leukemia relapsed and it is growing very rapidly. They stopped the boosting meds because it apparently only boosted the bad cells. So by now she has 72% abnormal cells and only 28% donor cells left even though a month ago she had 100% donor cells and everything was going to be uphill from then on so I thought. Jasmina saw my bloodshot eyes and told me "mama, no reason to cry... just think about something beautiful"!!! She always knows how to make me feel better and this is why we tell each other daily, "you are my MFEO". (Made For Each Other) In the meantime, the white of her eyes became yellow, indicating serious liver malfunctions. Her skin is blotchy, her urine so dark that you think someone threw a pot of coffee down the toilet and her stool is white. Wednesday they would have more results. So Wednesday came and her counts were even lower. Her energy a little bit back from the organic veggies (I hope) I was shooting three times a day in her tummy. So the doctors sat down with me and my dear friend Karen came to be the extra set of ears. Two choices - A low dose chemo to maintain her counts as they are so we could do a heavy duty chemo when she is six months post transplant - Or taking her of the medications, let her eat whatever she wants and go to Disney world to let her have fun in her last days. Well. I am not ready to give up after all we had thus far accomplished so I made an appointment with Dr. Carroll who was our first specialist back in NYU. Jasmina meanwhile received again a transfusion, more blood work etc. Since my faith in Dr. Carrol is beyond I can ever describe, and I call him Dr. Caring i/o Carrol, I will go with anything he can think of. Everything will be experimental from now on. He talked about an Epi Genetic protocol to re-program bad cells that has been very successful with adults, never children. So of course I think, well at some point there was a first adult if you get my drift. So to make a long story short, we had a very pleasant weekend at home and are now back inpatient at NYU. Yesterday she received platelets. Today she had another ultra sound of her liver and needed a skin biopsy to determine if the discoloration is caused by leukemia or Graft versus Host disease. By now the red blotchiness has darkened and a rash developed on her hands, knees and feet. Her eyes so yellow that they look fluorescent green, her tears are yellow, and her skin has an orange undertone like you see in bad make-up and the palms and bottom of her feet red. Her liver and spleen enlarged. When they took a skin biopsy today, she screamed in pain and the doctor told her that she was allowed to punch him after. When it was over I reminded her. She punched him and then somehow did not stop - letting out all her anger, all in perfect form from her Karate lessons pre-leukemia. Tight fist, straight wrist and letting the power come from her upper body. I was proud!! Tomorrow morning the gastro intestinal experts will check out her tummy. More test to follow. I know very well that her chances have decreased dramatically and a true miracle is needed at this point. So I keep hoping for a miracle despite some people that tell me that it might be time to let go. If that happens I know I need to do something drastic. Either someone PLEASE knock me into a coma for a while or immediately take in a bunch of foster kids. And then there are the obvious logistics. Many months ago my friend Mariana creatively located the birth family and we took a plane one Saturday morning to swab them in a last resort moment before a donor was found since I learned about a new treatment they can do with Hap-lo identities. These are half matches and I wanted to cover all my options in case we were unable to find an unrelated donor. We met the birth mother, the grand-parents, the uncles and all 5 half siblings. They are wonderful people hoping to meet Jasmina one day. I promised them that when all would be back to normal they could. Now that there is a significant chance that it might not. Mariana is contacting them and inviting them to New York. They have been praying for her since they became aware so it is only fair to grant them this wish. But now as you can imagine, all kind of scenarios play off in my head and there is very little I am able to think about. I get so many well meaning mails/call from some of you but the truth is, I do not know my schedule next Wednesday. I do not know what I want to eat. I do not know how I hold up. What I do know is the following; I will keep fighting and hoping for a miracle. I know how to liquefy a whole chicken. I know how to sterilize syringes, medicine cups, pill splitters, the feeding tube extension etc. I know how to manage all her 16 medications (my kitchen counter looks like a pharmacy) and how to split, pulverize, mix and measure, keeping track of time to administer the different meds, how many and how much time in between. But I simply cannot make decisions for all the well meaning friends. As Karen said last Friday in a CB update, if you want to do something, please do but please do not ask. Some great things happened also last week. My friend Mike took me to the movies and held my hand for the entire time. The large lady with the sweet face whose name I don't even know, who took me in her arms and let me cry. My friend Gisela who without asking what I needed, stocked my fridge. Jasmina's best friend Isabelle who continues to be able to make her giggle like a, well..6 -year old. My friend Vanessa who genuinely told me last week Monday after the first bad news that (since I was obviously emotionally distraught) she'd drive me upstate that evening and take the bus back in the morning. I had to go back because I left my mom there and needed to bring her to the airport the following afternoon. Now we cannot go anymore because Jasmina is again ultra neutrophenic and extremely susceptible to infections. Her white count is 0.1 same as after radiation. My friend Elaine, who came over on Saturday, totally ignored me and baked cookies with Jasmina. This was a real treat for her because for those of you who know me well, I do not bake. I make things but do not bake things. My friend Carie, a student doctor we befriended who came over and let Jasmina give her a make- over with the huge amount of make- up Rihanna had given her. She left that evening with orange cheeks, an abundance of green eye-shadow and a bindi on her forehead on her way to meet her parents for dinner. Our friend Karen who just stops by and entertains Jasmina - My friend Jenny who works at Mac cosmetics and left a giant bag of goodies, courtesy of the Mac girls in front of the door. Bracha, Jasmina's favorite nurse who stopped by in the hospital, making Jasmina smile from ear to ear. My boss, who more than generously continues to give me a break from the office even though by law, they are only obligated to grant FMLA for one month a year. The black cotton foundation who will give Jasmina the Dr. Betty Shabazz youth award because Jasmina has been such an inspiration to the community. DKMS, who wants to give Jasmina an award next year for having raised such great awareness concerning bone marrow donors. I thank my friend Billy who wrote Jasmina a postcard every day for the last eight months and flew over from Amsterdam this week to assist me in this difficult ordeal. I appreciate all my amazing and wonderful friends who I was able to count on and have stood by me this entire time. And then of course all the encouraging, sweet, much needed and appreciated messages I find on Caring Bridge. Some from people I never have met. I just want to say, thank you all so much from the bottom of my heart and please do NOT give up yet. Let's all keep hoping for that miracle.

Friday, November 6, 2009

I don't want to write this entry because I feel like I'm just dreaming and I'm afraid I will wake up as soon as I hit the SAVE button, but I have to tell you that the results of Jasmina's bone marrow and liver biopsies came back today and according to her doctors, there is NO leukemia in her bone marrow or liver....0%, none, nilly, void, gone, undetectable, miraculous!!!!!!!!!!!!!! Her liver malfunction is caused by the graft vs. host disease. So now we just need to get the graft vs. host and her liver better. There is no need for the experimental gene therapy and possibly no need for any future "aggressive" chemo treatments to cure the leukemia. They will alter her G vs. H meds to try and improve her liver function now that they know that is definitely what is causing the problem. As you can imagine, Thea is beside herself with "reserved" joy and disbelief. Tomorrow night Jasmina will be honored by the Black Cotton Foundation at their gala in Harlem. It will be a grand affair and we are very proud that they are honoring Jasmina. O.K., I'm going to hit the save button now so this will become the official, miraculous news! Sweet dreams.

Tuesday, November 10, 2009

Okay, this weekend has been great!!! First,- the emotional roller coaster. A month ago I had funeral visions when her leukemia was 72%. Finishing her princess winter wonderland room in the attic upstate and praying that she would be able to see it and live a fantasy at least once before she would deteriorate further in cancerland. Now that the leukemia is 0%, I can smile again and fantasize once more about a great future ahead.

But now, the exiting news. We are going to THE white house over Thanksgiving. A friend of mine contacted the "make a wish" foundation back in February and since Jasmina's leukemia was diagnosed the exact same day as the president's inauguration, ( I remember the nurses and doctors hovering over her doing all sorts of tests while watching Obama's big moment on TV) she decided she wants to meet Obama.

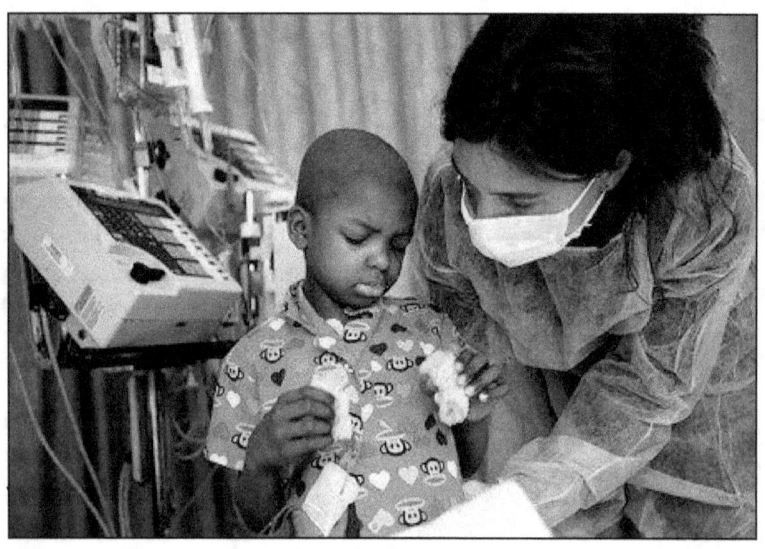

We will meet the President on Wednesday. Jasmina is going to give him a framed picture of her motivational "transplant" dress, I made for her from a tee-shirt that says "we can do it" with Michele Obama's face on it, she wore when she received her transplant on June 11.

I will of course slip Michelle some festive fabulous outfits from the company I work for. Jasmina is incredibly exited to meet him and fascinated that the White house has 132 rooms, 35 bathrooms and the fact that Obama had a pet monkey named "TATA" when he was her age. She is working on a list with questions, which has to be checked by security first.

We arrived in DC and were taken by limo to the hotel. I woke her up for her 6 AM medicine in the morning and all was fine. I let her sleep a bit more for the big moment ahead and was on the other side of the room ironing both of our White House outfits when she started complaining about pain at the site of her feeding tube. So once again, I removed the d... thing. This time a huge amount of gas escaped unlike the volcano-like tummy content a few weeks earlier. She felt better. Then moments later she cried in pain again and I called the lady who was waiting for us in the lobby if we could be a half hour late but she told me that the white house is on a very tight schedule. (-of course they are- what was I thinking?!!!)

At this point Jasmina's speech became incoherent and she had pain in her heart. She also wet the bed which is unusual. Then her eyes became unfocused. I pressed the alarm button of the hotel phone and then everything went really fast. The hotel security and Ambulance staff were phenomenal and we could not have lost many seconds. She was not breathing on her own and they put her on oxygen immediately. Then they asked her to open her mouth. By this time having been so long in the hospital, Jasmina can do this in her sleep but when she did not comply and I saw that her teeth were clenched, you know. Something was REALLY wrong.

In the ER, about 15 doctors, nurses hovered over her tiny body, putting tubes and IV's all over the place. Frantically I called Dr. Carroll in NY who knows the doctors here. All came over, post transplant doctor, neurology, oncology etc. - Including the VP of oncology who happens to be Dutch. We were in good hands. After many tests and more tests, the conclusion was that she developed PRES. Posterior Reversible Encephalopathy syndrome. The first word that stuck to me was "REVERSIBLE!!!" This PRES is due to one of the medications, Tacrolimus (why did no one ever tell me about this side effect???) and causes swelling in the white part of the brain (I saw it myself on the brain MRI). This together with her high blood pressure caused a seizure. The worst went through my head. Brain aneurysm, blood clot, brain dead, vegetable, etc.

So there we are in the emergency room with a social worker on one side of me and a priest on my other side and I am thinking, it was not supposed to go like this. I was supposed to make an attempt to pinch the president at this very moment. (or at least fantasize about doing so).

Later we were transferred to the ICU. There she was, just laying there for two days, out of it. She still has no recollection of these two days. A tube in her nose, her mouth attached to an incubator, in both of her hands and IV and her head attached to thousands of little wires to monitor more possible seizures. Her hands cuffed to the side of the bed like you see in movies about loony bins, so that she would not be able to tug one of the tubes. The white house called for an update and the president wanted to speak to me but I was in no mood to speak to anyone. I mean whatever can you say in a situation like this?

Then neurology, after studying the brain MRI, told me that she might have some brain damage and vision impairment thing going thru your mind is then, OKAY, not a vegetable, she will just need glasses.

The next morning she was able to follow commands like squeeze my hand etc. Also able to recognize how many fingers he doctor was holding up so they were very pleased with her progress. Later that day when Jasmina woke up, the first thing she said ( well not said, because she was still not breathing on her own and was not able to talk with the fat tube in her mouth, taped to her face), she wrote down; "How come it is Friday already?" The second sentence; "What happened to Obama?" At first she did not believe me that it was Friday and was angry. Then in no time her attitude was back and she was playing her DS. That's my girl. !!!!! It would not be Jasmina if she did not get out of this. She clearly is not brain damaged and has no impaired vision, HOORAY !!!!

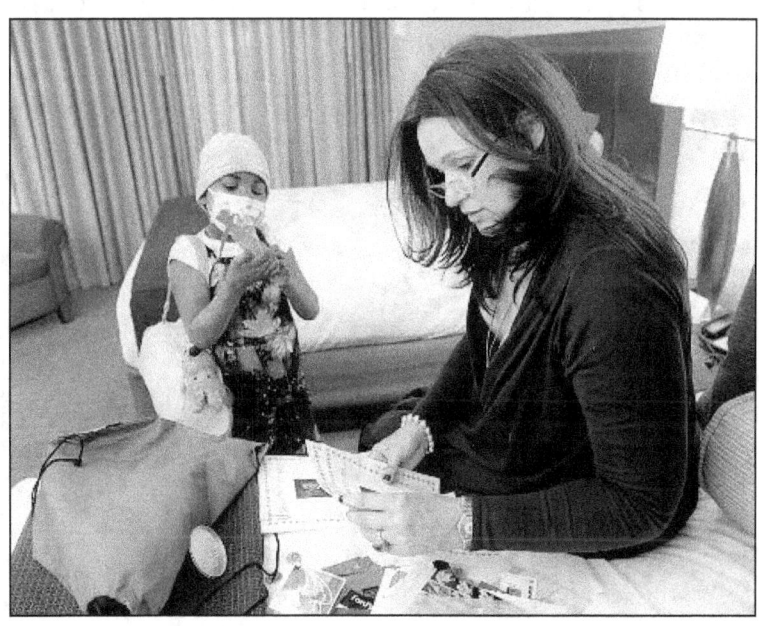

Later the same day I received a call that the white house was going to call me between 5.30 and 6.30 PM and that it would show up on my phone as "unknown".
The call came at 5.05 PM. I of course was not sure since the call came early and on top of that I rightfully presumed that a

representative would verify my name and put me "through", so I said, "who's this?". And there it was......."this is Barack Obama" in the nicest sexiest voice you can imagine. I wanted to say, "Say it again- PLEASE." but was able to contain my excitement ( the president has my cell number, how cool is that?) so we chatted a bit. He asked all about Jasmina's condition, recovery etc, and I thanked him for the opportunity. He asked if she was resting and unfortunately, she was sound asleep and I could not wake her up. So he said that when she is up to it, to call his office and he will talk to her. Jasmina is extremely disappointed that she did not meet him. The wonderful people at the "make a wish" foundation assured me that it will be rescheduled for a later date so that made her smile again.

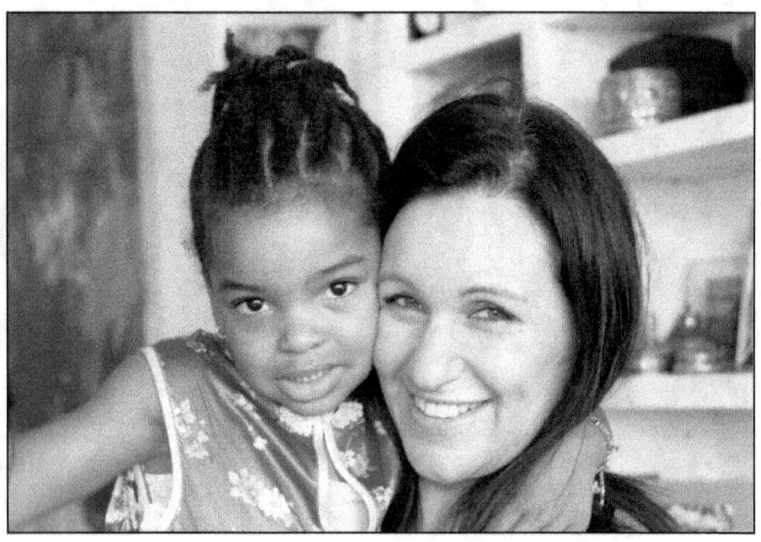

Sunday, December 6, 2009 1:37 PM, CST

From Thea. Jasmina's last tube came out on Wednesday. The evening before I had received a phone call that she might meet the president after all but I had to keep this a top secret. Somehow my phone stopped working too. I like to believe secret service had something to do with it preventing me from twitting a tweet but who knows. The next morning after the daily blood labs came in, she needed a blood transfusion. This takes time and I thought, oh well, it is never going to happen. Then the hospital PR lady knew about it and made the doctors run the transfusion at a faster speed since 2 PM, the limo would be there to pick us up and bring us to the white house. This is when I told Jasmina. She smiled from ear to ear. Sooo HAPPY!!!!

So off we went. Security is tight. Dogs came sniffing the limo and at every check point I needed again to show ID. Once we were in, it was fantastic. Somehow everyone knew her by name. Greeting her and smiling endearingly. They treated her like a VIP. We had to enter through the back because Oprah was shooting her Christmas special in the front of the White House. They showed Jasmina an assortment of Christmas trees. There are 34 of them in the white house - Including, a wish cardboard tree. People write a note and put this in the tree, much like the wish wall in Israel. She wrote, "I wish NO ONE will ever have leukemia anymore", rolled it up and stuck it in the tree. When we reached the waiting room of the Oval office, the door swung open and there he was. "Jasmina it is soooo nice to meet you" he said. She and I were led in. Barack carried her Hello Kitty IV fluid bag she was attached to. I stepped back and let them have their moment. They chatted about books, Christmas, first grade etc. I did not even realize that we were in the Oval office but apparently this is a big deal I am told. He asked her what she would like for Christmas and she promptly answered,- a violin. (!!!) This was mentioned in the NY Daily News a few days ago resulting in three offers of people who want to donate a violin. (Today, Sunday, a man and his wife came over and presented her with a brand new beautiful violin. Now I have to find a teacher)

Jasmina meets President Barack Obama

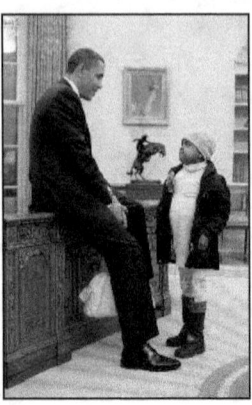

He was extremely compassionate and sweet with her-
Complimenting her on her maturity and articulation. When
it was time to leave he said, "Come here and give me a
hug". Now mind you, I am still watching this scenario from
a few feet distance but was not letting a chance like this go
by, so I said; "Excuse me? How about a picture with the
three of us?" The fact that he made time for her was
unbelievably amazing and it is a truly magical experience
she will never forget. He also told her that if there was
anything she needed to let him know and that she could
always write to him. She will be able to do this through the
wonderful people at "make a wish". The two packages with
gifts we brought had to be left with secret service. I hope
he will get them.

Jasmina has now a really swollen tummy, her face blown up from
the steroids and another side effect of one of the medications,
excessive hair growth. Her temples and forehead are covered in

black fuzz. Later she told the security guard that she could not wait to tell her best friend. The security guard said, "oh Isabelle, the girl in the video!!" Everyone seems to know these two. Later in the hotel she kept making drawings of Obama and the next morning told me that she dreamed about him.

Next week she will get another bone marrow biopsy. Hopefully she will still be in remission.

Wednesday, January 27, 2010 10:22 PM, CST

Today, January 27th, at 10:55 p.m. Jasmina lost her fight against leukeamia.

www.oneforjasmina.com

# THE MATCH

Ajani's Story

In Nigeria, "Ajani" means "he who wins the struggle." In Roanoke, Virginia, it means the same thing. Ajani was diagnosed with leukemia three years ago at age two. His doctor gave him three months to live, unless he got an unrelated umbilical cord blood transplant. Fortunately, a matching cord blood unit was found, thanks to another family's generous decision to donate their baby's' cord blood to a public cord blood bank.

Ajani received his transplant at Duke University Hospital, and his mother Risa has been trying to keep up with him ever since. This is no small task, since Ajani's motor is always running. He enjoys riding his bike, playing ball of any kind, listening to music and competing with his cousins in just about anything

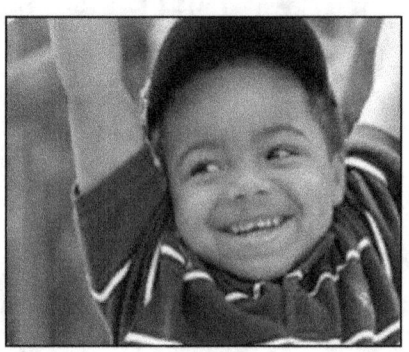

Ajani

"No question, the transplant saved my son's life," says Risa. "I thought I appreciated him before, but after all he's gone through, I appreciate him even more now." In Edo, one of the languages of Nigeria, Ajani means "he who wins the struggle." Ajani is living up to his name in every way.

My Stem Cell Donation Story

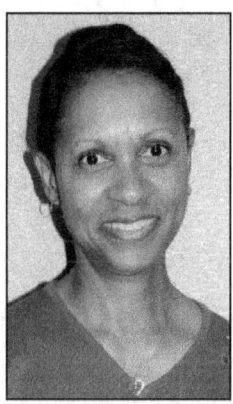

Patricia Peoples Smith

Two-thousand-seven was a trying year for me. It began with an unexpected health decline of my 93 year old father, which led to numerous trips between Atlanta and Virginia, conference calls with my brothers, and continuous on-the-spot decisions about hospitals, rehab, in-home care, and nursing homes. September of that year found me overwhelmed, overworked, sad, and feeling somewhat useless. It was at that time that I received a solicitor-sounding message on my home phone. I quickly deleted it, only to discover a similar message on my cell phone. As I listened closely to the words, my suspicious nature quickly dissipated and was replaced with excitement. Someone was calling from the National Marrow Donor Program (NMDP), and I was a potential match for someone in need!

I quickly returned the call, and that began my relationship with a host of people dedicated to connecting life-givers with life-strugglers. The coordinator in Charlotte, NC, Calesta Tyson, began to unfold the world of bone marrow and stem cell transplantation to me in a concise and non-threatening manner. She could hardly finish answering one of my questions before I was asking another. I wanted to know all about the procedure, but I mainly wanted to know about the person, the one who needed help. She informed me that because of privacy laws, the only information I could be given was the fact that it was a 41-year-old African-American female with leukemia. I didn't have a name or a face, but I immediately had a "soul" connection with someone somewhere in the world whose health could possibly be radically transformed with just a little bit of life inside of me, and that was GOOD NEWS!

My connection with NMDP (now "Be The Match") began in 1986 when a young girl in my church community was diagnosed with leukemia. I don't remember the specifics; only that she needed a donor match in order to receive bone marrow. I remember going to the donor drive held at our church and hearing the presenter share the sad reality that while the best matches come from within one's race, there were only a few African-Americans on the Registry. My immediate unconscious response was, "That's ridiculous!" Hence, I did not hesitate to have a tiny bit of blood drawn and submitted to (what I call) an international registry of hope. (Sadly, the little girl never found a match and passed away.)

As I chatted with Calesta in the ensuing months, I learned that the process of donating was quite simple. I went to a local laboratory (convenient to my home and work) to have a few blood samples drawn for further analysis. The young lady's physician would review the results and in eight to ten weeks make a decision regarding whether I was a good match for his patient. After the blood was drawn, I returned to my routine of caring for my father long-distance, while working fulltime as an occupational therapist in a school system. All awhile, I was mentally counting down those eight-to-ten weeks

Needless to say, I was ecstatic when I returned home one day and found a message from Calesta asking me to call her right away. The return of that call started a wave of events which encouraged me greatly at a time when I needed it most. A packet of material was shipped to me, which included a video explaining the bone marrow and stem cell transplants. I jotted my questions as I watched the tape, eager to know all about the procedure that I WITHOUT QUESTION would agree to be apart of. Calesta phoned me after I had a chance to review all of the materials. Having used most of my sick leave to care for my father, I decided to donate stem cells since it would require less time from work and some of the research suggested that stem cell recipients seemed to fair better than bone marrow recipients.

I was thoroughly impressed with the ease in which the National Organization's office coordinated their efforts with the collection hospital to schedule all of the medical procedures. They made every effort to accommodate my schedule while fulfilling the medical needs of the patient in a timely manner. I spent the day at a local Atlanta hospital undergoing a complete physical (including lunch and parking!) At the end of the day, the presiding physician entered the room and asked me if I still "wanted to do this?" I jubilantly responded, "Absolutely!"

The next few weeks were marked with more frequent correspondence from Calesta, once informing me that the patient had had a setback and the scheduled stem cell collection would have to be delayed until she was more physically stable. As the rescheduled date approached, I was reminded that the few weeks prior to the collection were crucial. While this was the time in which I was vigilant about getting my rest, maintaining my state of wellness, and running from anyone who *looked* like they were about to cough, I knew that the young woman was slowly having her bone marrow and immune system destroyed so that she could receive my cells. I knew that should I choose to back out now, her death was imminent. This thought never crossed my mind; in fact, my mind was made up in 1986 when I entered the Registry.

In mid-December the preliminaries had been taken care of, the patient was prepped for the procedure, and the collection day/s was scheduled. I had made an earlier visit to the hospital wing where the collections would be taken. The nursing staff was kind, caring, and congratulatory. They carefully checked my veins to decide whether there appeared to be viable ones that could sustain the 3-4 hour procedure. One arm was questionable, but the Head Nurse felt that there were several veins to choose from.

Five days prior to the collection, I began receiving a painless injection of a drug that was designed to pull the stem cells from the bone marrow into the bloodstream for easier collection. The nursing staff explained the potential side effects of the drug, but my only symptoms were an occasional back or hip spasm. It did not interfere with my job nor incapacitate me in the least.

The national organization provided hotel accommodations close to the hospital, which allowed for two restful nights away from home, minimal travel time, and valet parking at the hospital. The nurses informed me of each step of the process, making sure that I was comfortable. There was a brief tense moment when my left arm proved to only have one viable vein through which my ten units of blood would pass. If it collapsed during the collection I would have to be admitted and have a port surgically inserted. However, each day's collection took about 3 ½ hours and that little David-size vein withstood the pressure of Goliath-size amounts of blood forcing its way through. You may wonder what I was doing the entire time of the procedure. I was draped in a hospital gown, fluffed with soft pillows, and covered with just the amount of blankets. I laid in a semi-reclined position in a regular hospital bed right across from the nurse's station where they checked on me frequently. The time was mainly spent chatting about the joys of having person after person come to donate their cells. When we were not chatting, I was allowed to watch cable television. On the first collection day, another coordinator from the Charlotte office made a visit. She was in town to personally oversee the shipping of the collected stem cells. She also presented me with an engraved clock as an expression of gratitude. Since she was also staying in the same hotel as I, we had an opportunity to have dinner together and I was given the opportunity to hear how rewarding her job was and how impactful the National Registry had been in the lives of countless thousands. I returned to work the day after the collection was completed, but my follow up did not end. Calesta continued to monitor my progress and made sure that I was not having any adverse reactions to the procedure. She also informed me that the recipient was responding well to the donation. That was the best Christmas gift I could have been given.

Once a year's time had passed, I began to get that antsy feeling again. I had not forgotten that the original material from the Registry mentioned that the donor and recipient could share personal information after one year. I still remember that day in early-Spring of 2009 when I received a call from the City of Hope Cancer Center in LA, inviting me to their annual Bone Marrow Transplant Reunion. I, once again, was treated like royalty, when a friend and I were flown to California, lavished with state of the art hotel accommodations, and given the privilege to be united with my recipient, Catherine Fuller, in front of hundreds of former donors, recipients, hospital staff, and friends. She and her family were abundantly grateful for my gift of stem cells, and I in turn was grateful to witness what a few bags of blood could do for another's life. I often recall how Catherine's sixteen-year-old daughter hovered near me that day, as if it were her way of saying "because of you I have my mother." One of Catherine's sisters, however, shared some information that cast a shadow over the entire event. She mentioned that there were 22 people on the Registry who had been contacted about being a potential match for Catherine...and they all said NO. My response was the same as that in 1986: "That's ridiculous". And this is why I share my story with you. While I have had good health most of my 52 years, I recognize that that could change in a moment's notice. It would sadden me to know that someone had the privilege to give me life-saving blood and refused to even try. I tend to believe that the manner in which you treat people will be returned to you, so I aspire to do the right thing by others, no matter their race. I hope that my story will inspire many to do the same, and to become a part of this wonderful Registry of hope.

Catherine Fuller the recipient

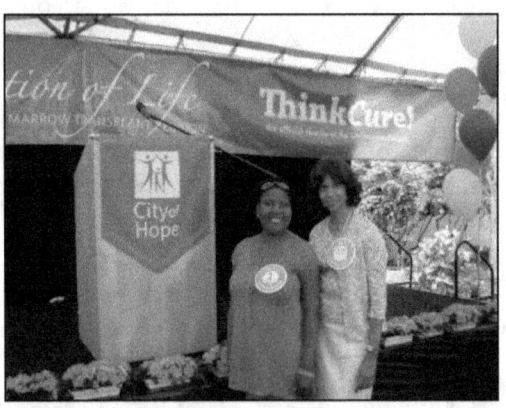

Donor Pat Smith and recipient Catherine Fuller

## Catherine Fuller

"I have two children, a son, 22 and a daughter aged 17."

"I was working as a nurse when I was diagnosed with AML on March 30 2007. I had a trip to Las Vegas planned in a couple of weeks, and my initial reaction when I got diagnosed was that fact that I was bummed that I would not be able to make it to Vegas."

"I had been having symptoms for a long time but I just kept ignoring them. It got so bad that I could not walk more than 20 steps without becoming very fatigued. When that went on for a month or so I knew I had to go to the doctor."

"I was diagnosed on a Friday and went to Cedars (Hospital?) where I asked a nurse if I could wait a couple of weeks before going to the hospital. She looked at me as if I were a crazy person and advised me to go as soon as possible."

"I worked as nurse and I saw children with cancer and had taken care of them. They always seemed happy and were running around like little children, the only difference was that they had bald heads, so I never saw my leukemia diagnosis as anything but an inconvenience."

"I needed a bone marrow match from the very beginning, and they started a search for me from the start. I had donor drives held for me and the search for my match started in August of 2007. I found 20 possible matches and they all said no. In October of 2007 they found Pat Peoples Smith to be a potential match and she said 'yes', she would do it."

"My reaction to 20 people saying no was one of confusion. Why would people put themselves on the list if they did not intend on donating?"

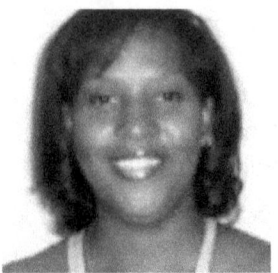
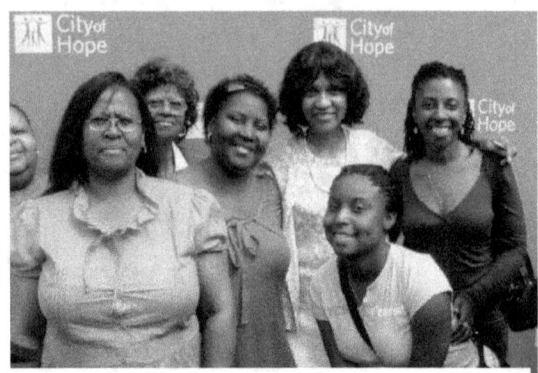

Catherine Fuller with her family and Pat Smith

I have 9 siblings who were all tested and none of them were a match for me. 8 of us have both the same mother and father, and not one sibling was a match.

"I was happy and relieved when they found Pat and she agreed to go through the process. I had the transplant December 13 2007 at 11:55 PM. After the transplant, the first time the doctors tested my blood they still saw some of my bone marrow, but the second time they tested my blood they found all donor cells – that meant the leukemia was gone."

"My reaction to meeting my donor was the fact that I was grateful for what she had done for me. She had the same blood type as me we were both O positive. I got to meet her a year after the transplant, and I was just grateful that I would be able to see my children grow up and have children of their own."

"It's a small bit of your time and efforts to give someone else back their life. How many opportunities do you get to save a life? I am definitely for people joining the registry."

*If you are between the age of 18 and 60, in reasonably good health*
*You can join the "Be the Match" registry.*

*If we do not step up to the plate and join the registry*
*Who will be there to help save someone's life?*

# Conclusion

The numbers regarding the disparity in health care are astounding, overwhelming and appalling. And yet, it is not about numbers. It is about every person suffering with life-threatening disease such as leukemia and sickle cell. It is about the families anxiously waiting around hospital beds watching loved ones in pain and distress. It is about the 86 percent of Blacks in need of a transplant they will never receive. It is about the thousands who have made their transition too soon and left to many behind. It is about their unfinished works and unfulfilled dreams and aspirations. It is about the loved ones that still carry them in their heart and care for the children and siblings they left behind. It is about the children that watched their parent or sibling slip away and wondered why? It is about the parents and grand- parents that watched their offspring fight until their strength and energy was exhausted. It is about the disappointments when potential donors simply walked away and said, "I changed my mind." It is about the health care providers who exhaust all their energy, strength and resources only to walk into a room and see the empty bed. It is about those who search sites world-wide and find hundreds of matches for Caucasians and next to none for an African American. It is about someone, lying in a hospital bed and hoping that someone like you will step forward and be the one they need to give them hope, as they are, *In Search of a Match.*

.

# FACTS
# AND
# STATS

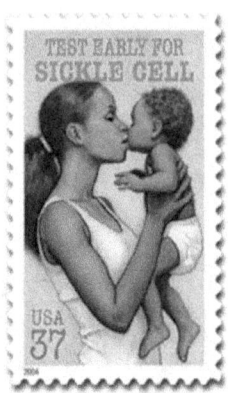

In 2004 the Sickle Cell Disease Awareness Stamp was created raising public awareness of health and social issues. The inscription "Test Early for Sickle Cell" conveys the importance of early testing.

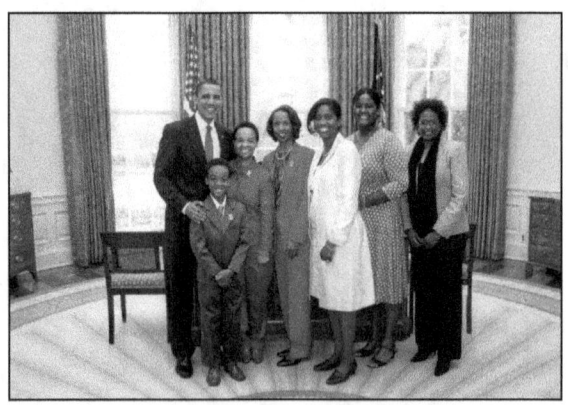

President Barack Obama meets with
Sickle Cell Disease Association of America

## Sickle Cell Disease and the Sickle Cell Trait

Sickle cell disease has been known to the peoples of Africa for hundreds of years. In West Africa various ethnic groups gave the condition different names:

- Ga tribe: CHwechweechwe
- Faute tribe: Nwiiwii
- Ewe tribe: Nuidudui
- Twi tribe: Ahotutuo

*The repeated syllables are said to mimic the cries of the children suffering from the disease.*

- A history of the condition tracked reports back to 1670 in one Ghanaian family.
- In the US in 1846, a paper entitled "Case of Absence of the Spleen" (from the *Southern Journal of Medical Pharmacology*), was probably the first to describe sickle cell disease. It discussed the case of a runaway slave who had been executed. His body was autopsied and found to have "the strange phenomenon of a man having lived without a spleen." Although the slave's condition was typical, the doctor had no way of knowing this as the disease had not yet been "discovered."
- The African medical literature reported this condition in the 1870s, where it was known locally as **ogbanjes** ("children who come and go") because of the very high infant mortality rate caused by this condition.
- The first formal report of sickle cell disease came out of Chicago about 50 years later, in 1910 when a patient of his from the West Indies had an anemia characterized by unusual red cells that were "sickle shaped.
- In 1922, after three more cases were reported, the disease was named "sickle cell anemia.

- In 1948, using the new technique of protein electrophoresis, Linus Pauling and Harvey Itano showed that the hemoglobin from patients with sickle cell disease is different than that of others. This made sickle cell disease the first disorder in which an abnormality in a protein was known to be at fault

What is Sickle Cell Disease?
- It is a group of inherited red blood cell disorders
- It is the most common genetic disease in the US.
- *Normal red blood cells are round like doughnuts, and they move through small blood tubes in the body to deliver oxygen. Sickle red blood cells become hard, sticky and shaped like sickles used to cut wheat. When these hard and pointed red cells go through the small blood tube, they clog the flow and break apart. This can cause pain, damage and a low blood count, or anemia.*

What makes the red cell sickle?

- There is a substance in the red cell called hemoglobin that carries oxygen inside the cell. One little change in this substance causes the hemoglobin to form long rods in the red cell when it gives away oxygen. These rigid rods change the red cell into a sickle shape.

How do you get Sickle Cell?

- You inherit the abnormal hemoglobin from both parents who may be carriers with sickle cell trait or parents with sickle cell disease.
- About 2.5 million African-Americans (1 in 12) are carriers (AS) of the sickle cell trait. People who are carriers may not even be aware that they are carrying the S allele!

A cure for Sickle Cell Disease

- In **1984**, bone marrow transplantation in a child with sickle cell disease produced the first reported cure of the disease. The transplantation was done to treat acute leukemia. The child's sickle cell disease was cured as a side-event. The procedure nonetheless set the precedence for efforts directed specifically at sickle cell disease.

Sickle Cell Disease and Malaria
- It is now known that, when invaded by the malarial parasite, normally stable red cells of someone with the sickle cell trait can sickle in a low oxygen environment (like the veins). The sickling process destroys the invading organism and prevents it from spreading through the body.
- In regions repeatedly devastated by malaria, people who carry the sickle cell trait will have a greater chance for survival than other individuals.
- Only those with sickle cell trait, not the disease, are protected against malaria.

### Bone Marrow Transplant for Sickle cell patients

There are several hundred children worldwide that have been cured with a bone marrow transplant. The risk of death factor is about 8%. The procedure takes several months and usually requires a brother or sister with a HLA match. The cost is approximately$250,000.

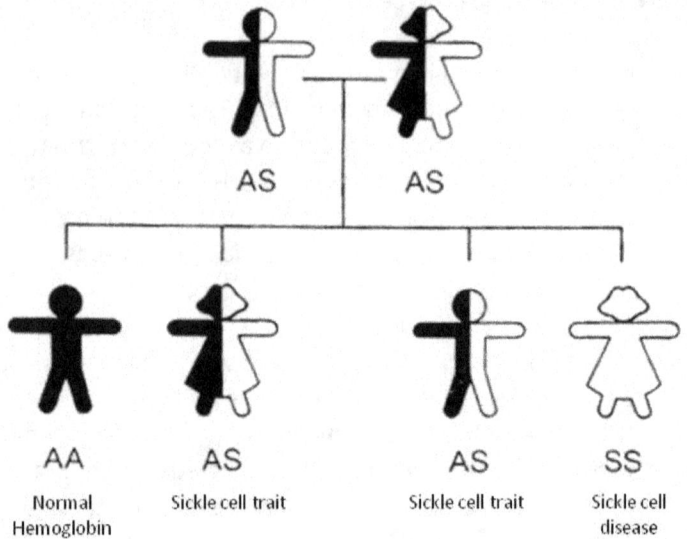

| AA | AS | AS | SS |
|---|---|---|---|
| Normal Hemoglobin | Sickle cell trait | Sickle cell trait | Sickle cell disease |

If both parents have the sickle cell trait (S) the chances are one in four that the child may be born with sickle cell disease.

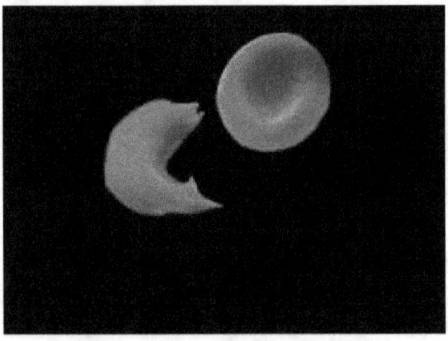

Normal and sickle cell

### Leukemia

Leukemia is really a word that describes a group of diseases that are cancers of the blood and bone marrow. The leukemia's vary a great deal in how they act—from fast acting to slow growing.

The name given to fast acting leukemia is "acute". Leukemia is called "chronic" when the disease acts slower.

There are two major types of white blood cells that become cancerous. These are either myeloid or lymphocytic. Myeloid refers to the type of white cell that is important in killing bacteria (germs). Lymphocytic cells are the white cells that have a broad role in immunity.

The four most common types of adult leukemia are:

- Acute lymphocytic leukemia
- Acute myeloid leukemia
- Chronic lymphocytic leukemia
- Chronic myeloid leukemia

**Who Gets Leukemia?**

- Many times the cause of leukemia is not known. Anyone at any age can get leukemia.

**What Are the Symptoms of Leukemia?**

The symptoms of acute leukemia appear and get worse quickly. In chronic leukemia, symptoms may not appear for a long time. When they do appear, they usually are mild at first and get worse slowly. Many times chronic leukemia is found during a routine check-up.

Some of the common symptoms of leukemia are:

- Fever, chills or flu-like symptoms
- Night sweats
- Weakness and tiredness

- Easy bleeding or bruising
- Tiny red spots under the skin
- Swollen or bleeding gums
- Nights sweats
- Swollen lymph glands

Blood & Marrow Transplantation–patients who have a BMT will face an increased risk of infection, bleeding and other side effects of the large doses of chemotherapy and radiation. Graft versus host disease (GVHD) may occur in patients who receive bone marrow from a donor. In GVHD, the donated marrow reacts against the patient's tissues (most often the liver, skin and the digestive tract). GVHD can be mild or very severe. It can occur any time after the transplant–even years later. Drugs may be given to reduce the risk of GVHD and to treat the problem if it occurs.

Someone once described leukemia as a "liquid tumor."

How do you fare "In Search of a Match?

According to the National Marrow Donor Program:

Theoretical Probability of Patient's finding at least One matched donor by racial and ethnic Group
Recent estimates of this based on the registry as of Jan 1, 2008 provide the following race breakdown of an 8/8 allele ("full") matched donor
> African American: 18.8%
> Asian/Pacific Islander: 27.6%
> European American: 57.3%
> Hispanic or Latino:  34.3%

Recent estimates of the probability of finding a 7/8 allele match rate, which is often a clinically acceptable donor match provides the breakdown range:
> African American: 60-80%
> Asian/Pacific Islander: 60-80%
> European American:  85-95%
> Hispanic or Latino: 70-85%

### Total Transplant Recipients By Race and Ethnicity

| | |
|---|---|
| Black or African American | 800 |
| American Indian/Alaska Native | 83 |
| Asian | More than 500 |
| Native Hawaiian or other Pacific Islander | 17 |
| White | More than 16,000 |
| Hispanic/other/unknown | More than 2,100 |
| **Total** | More than 20,000 |

83% of African American patients do not receive a life saving transplant.

## RESOURCES and web sites

**A Bone Marrow Wish**
www.bonemarrowwish.org
**Be The Match**
www.bethematch.org
**Be Transfusion Smart**
www.betransfusionsmart.com
**Black Bone Marrow**
www.blackbonemarrow.com
**BMDI BMT Support Group**
www.fightcancer.org
**BMT Support**
www.BMTsupport.org
**CML Earth**
www.cmlearth.com
**Daily Strength (BMT Support Group)**
www.dailystrength.org/
**DKMS Americas**
www.dkmsamericas.org
**HBCU Be The Match Registry**
www.hbcu.bethematch.org
**Marrow For Life**
www.marrowforlife.org
**National Marrow Donor Program**
www.nmdp.org
**National Minority Organ and Tissue Transplant
Education Program**
www.nationalmottep.org
**NMDP Transplant Links**
www.nbmtlink.org/web_links.htm
**Preserve Our Legacy, Inc.**
www.preserveourlegacy.org
**Save A Life Network**
www.savealifenetwork.org
**Stemcyte**
www.stemcytefamily.com

## LEUKEMIA
**African Carribbean Leukemia Trust**
www.aclt.org
**Greek Gray Leukemia Foundation**
www.gglf.org

**One For Jasmina**
www.oneforjasmina.com
**Brla T. Chism Foundation**
www.BriaTChism.org
**Caring Bridge**
www.caringbridge.org
**Jes Us 4 Jackie**
www.jesus4jackie.com
**Gift of Life Campaign**
www.giftoflifeonline.org

**Jaden's Law**

www.jadenslaw.org

**SICKLE CELL DISEASE:**
**About Sickle Cell Disease**
www.sicklecellinfo.net
**American Sickle Cell Anemia Association (ASCAA)**
www.ascaa.org
**Children's Healthcare of Atlanta**
www.choa.org/hemonc/sickle.shtml
**Comprehensive Sickle Cell Centers**
www.rhofed.com/sickle/Direct.htm
**Coulson Sickle Cell Foundation of Sierra Leone**
www.coulsonsicklecell.org
**Face Foundation**
www.facefoundationinc.org
**Health Reports**
www.Health-Reports.com/sicklecell
**Medical College of Georgia Sickle Cell Clinic**
www.mcg.edu/centers/sicklecell
**SCD Soldier Network**
www.scdsoldiernetwork.com
**Sickle Cell Disease Association of America**
www.sicklecelldisease.org
**Sickle Cell Foundation of Georgia**
www.sicklecellga.org
**Sickle Cell Information Center (Grady, Emory, Aflac, Morehouse)**
www.scinfo.org

**Sickle Cell Society**

www.sicklecellsociety.org

## A Special Tribute to Marrow For Life
### By The JamPoet

If I can give a portion of my life, yet still live to see the gift
I'd lift my hands and volunteer
I'd agree freely the opportunity to free me
Of my tears for the years
I've felt the families
Fear of losing their loved one
I'd mine my marrow like diamonds
A priceless miracle
I'd lay my reservations down at the feet of odds
Because I live by the grace of faith in my higher power
I am empowered to change someone's final hour
To infinite minutes of precious seconds of second chances
I have the power to stand on the summit of someone's
circumstances
And make heroic advances towards the reward of saving a life
I absorb all my lessons
And countless soul searching sessions
And proceed to act kindly
Taking every good deed in me
And unselfishly giving
A harvest of going against the grain
There's no pain id feel that would match
Someone's journey through this life altering disease
There's no pain id feel that would match
The many heart wrenching pleas
Families make time after time
In order to find and remind the races
That they are racing to spare a beloveds life
My sigh is a sign of last breaths and stolen moments
The pain and stress in ones chest
When endure is all they got left
We forget

Of all things out of our control
This isn't it
Each one that is eligible holds a miracle
In order to move you just need one
One daughter, one mother, one sister, one brother,
One loved one, husband, or wife
It's one deed, one match, one victory for life
What's painfully true is many will draw
Their last breath waiting on you
From this day forward I pay forward
The love for my community with my name on a registry
Too many times I think what if it were me
Too many times I didn't want to believe
There is a miracle waiting on me
My weight in miracle gold is me
I hold the key to life
The shortlist it's not long
The waiting list doesn't have long
The greatest gift you can give
Is affording someone a chance to live
They say all the world's a stage
And a hand extended to one in need
Is a hand that has been well played
When you are called to act
Are you moved or dissuade?
When it comes to Marrow for Life
Will you play it safe or will you save?
Register Today

*The JamPoet*

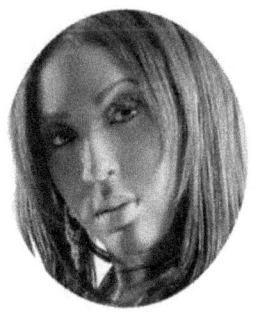